LIVELIFE365

LIVELIFE365

A Practical Self-Help Guide to Better Health, Nutrition, Weight Loss, Motivation, Personal Growth, and Life

Mike Foster

Creator of livelife365.com

CONTENTS

I.   Introduction: What is livelie365? pg. 11

II. Who Is Mike Foster? pg. 17

III. Healthy Lifestyle pg. 23

- Nutrition pg. 25
- Fitness pg. 93
- Weight Loss pg. 111

IV. Personal Development pg. 129

- Motivation pg. 131
- Inspiration pg. 165
- Balance pg. 193

V.   Entertainment pg. 205

- Humor pg. 207
- Opinion pg. 233
- Etc... pg. 257

VI. Feedback: livelife365 is working! Pg. 283

INTRODUCTION

I am sitting on the lanai at one of my favorite places in the world, staring out at the splendor that is the Pacific Ocean, mesmerized by the steady rumble of its soothing chants as it pounds its endless rhythmic beat into the shore of our Maui condo. This is where it all began, where the seed of the concept that was to become *livelife365* was born.

My name is Mike Foster. I have been enjoying and embracing life for more than half a century. I have had my share of ups and downs, like any other human being who has somehow survived fifty years on this planet. I've worked hard most of my life, and from the fruits of those arduous labors I have been fortunate enough to be able to afford a few perks that a steady paycheck and some fortuitous investments can create; like this timeshare condo my wife and I purchased a few years ago. I have also experienced my share of setbacks, heartbreaks, letdowns and meltdowns along the road to my almost mid-fifties, so many that I have dedicated an entire chapter of this book recounting them in painful detail.

But I'm not here to talk about my past just yet, not right now. Actually, right this second I am at peace with my world, happy and focused, healthy and fulfilled, content to kick back and watch the waves from a beachside condo in one of the most scenic places on earth, while reflecting on one of my most satisfying lifetime accomplishments:

LIVELIFE365

What is *livelife365*?

Well, *livelife365* is lots of things: a healthy philosophy about how to live your life to its fullest, every day in every way, while practicing an active, fit lifestyle; as well as a motivational, inspirational, personal development concept, that encourages learning from your mistakes while taking personal accountability for your actions…all done in an entertaining, and often humorous, way.

Livelife365 is one of the most popular self-help video websites on the Internet.

Livelife365 is a popular healthy lifestyle blog.

Livelife365 is funny song parodies, succinct commentaries about current events, a philosophical questioning about death and life, happiness and depression, weight loss and addictions, hobbies and helping others. *Life*.

Several year ago I was grossly overweight, had high blood pressure, dangerous cholesterol and glucose levels. I suffered from every type of gastrointestinal ailment: acid reflux, stomach pains, constipation, uncomfortable bloating; you name it.

To put it bluntly, I was slowly killing myself with my lifestyle. I was not only overweight and unhealthy; I was unhappy, depressed, and desperate for a change.

So I decided to do something about it. I figured out a way to change my life for the better.

- I researched, analyzed, learned, and changed my eating habits
- I consumed fewer calories, and made those calories that I did eat count
- I added more fiber to my diet: fruits, veggies, beans, nuts, whole grains
- I reduced my saturated fats, eliminating red meats, fried foods, cheese and processed foods.
- I increased my physical activities, worked out with weights and rode a stationary bike every other day. I also walked two miles every day
- I added natural supplements and non-synthetic multivitamins to my daily regimen
- I kept a journal of everything I consumed—everything!
- And I set goals, lots of goals, every day, every week, every month, until…

I LOST 40 POUNDS IN SIX MONTHS!

The changeover was as staggering and mind-opening as it was wonderful and exhilarating:

- I felt amazing
- I lowered my cholesterol, naturally, down to my healthiest levels in years
- I brought my blood pressure and glucose levels under control
- I stopped gobbling antacids like salted peanuts and eliminated all my gastrointestinal problems
- I felt ten years younger
- And I was so excited about all of the amazing changes that I was able to accomplish with my newfound lifestyle that I wanted to find a way to share them all with as many people as I possibly could. I wanted to be able to help others with my successes and positive results, help change their lives just like I was able to change mine.

Bringing me back to today, sitting here on my lanai, gazing serenely and contentedly out at the endless ocean, reflecting on the moment that changed my life, and hopefully will change yours, too.

I consider myself a blessed and lucky man—I have a wonderful wife, a happy, healthy, loving, and successful marriage, achieved from hard work and mutual respect. We also have been fortunate in that we have been able to earn decent livings, affording us the ability to lead fulfilled and rich lives. This, again, is the result of hard work, determined and focused planning and investing, allowing us the luxury of my being able to sit in this lounge chair and taking in this magnificent vista.

It was during one of these Maui sojourns, a time I use to decompress, reinvigorate, renew and revive my mind, body and spirit after months of arduous efforts and a grueling schedule of a demanding career, that inspiration struck. And like the man with an idea that he dreams will change the world, running through the streets shouting *"Eureka!"*, I, too, felt that twitch of something special, that tremble of excitement inside my bones that maybe I had something—a vision, a program, an idea, a way that I could share my successes, programs, visions, and philosophies—that could change the world.

So, after days of basking in the sun, enjoying long walks along the beach, dining out and chilling out on my favorite place in the world, I spent my evenings developing, designing, inventing and, finally, creating my website:

LIVELIFE365.COM

Returning to the mainland, the power of creative energy driving me, I sat down and hammered out the framework for my healthy living, personal development, and entertainment video website.

Several years, and hundreds and hundreds of videos, not to mention an equal amount of posts and articles, later, I had another *"Eureka!"* moment. I realized that while the Internet is big time stuff and reaches billions of people, it still does not reach everyone who needs to be reached. So I decided to go old school, and write this book, hoping to reach all those other folks out there, like yourself, who either do not surf the web or surf in cyber waters other than the ones my websites occupy.

Livelife365 has already reached hundreds of thousands of people in a relatively short period of time. The countless emails and letters I've received from site visitors, video watchers, and blog readers whom my programs and vision have helped and touched and changed is beyond my wildest dreams.

Yet, for me, that is not enough, merely the tip of the iceberg. Why? Because I still feel that I can reach more people who are looking for the little push, that one helpful tip or ah-ha moment, that thoughtful nudge in the right direction that will help them to change their lives for the better. Help them lose weight, eat right, improve their relationships, their self-confidence; inspire them to pick up a hobby or volunteer their time to a worthy cause. And, as important as all of the above, enjoy themselves and laugh along the way.

So it made perfect sense to go back to the place where it all started, back to that lanai (which, for those of you wondering, is just the Hawaiian word for patio) in that condo on that beach in Maui to put pen to paper and write this book that will, hopefully, change your life for the better. And with the overall desire to reach more people than I ever dreamed of reaching.

People, like you, who are perhaps searching for hope, help, direction, motivation, inspiration, education, entertainment, humor, happiness, all delivered with a proven formula and commonsense approach that can change the way you look at yourself, and your life.

Welcome to *livelife365*.

Over the next several pages I will offer you countless ways that will help you change your life, yes, for the better, but, really my message and goal is for you to start living your life every day in every way. Learn:

- Improve your Triad of Balance (Mind, Body, Spirit)
- Lose two pounds a week
- The key to weight loss
- What is Jicama?
- In Search of vegetable protein
- Healthy Snacking
- Do you believe?
- Is it just me?
- Drink green tea every day
- Just do it: 10 tips to get you started
- Count your calories, and make your calories count
- A life without goals is a life unfulfilled

    The list is endless…

Here is all I ask of you, someone, by the way, that I am already indebted to and inspired by (because you've already taken the first difficult step in purchasing this book):

ARE YOU READY TO CHANGE YOUR LIFE?

FOR THE BETTER?

I understand how difficult this task is, believe me, I do. I've been through some major changes in my life, and figure to go through a few more before my time on this planet is done. And I totally understand that you probably have a good idea of what you need to do with your life, that you, if you are like billions of other people, need to lose some weight, eat better, save more money, earn more money, improve your relationships, your outlook, yourself. But just because you know you need to change, doesn't make actually changing any easier. This book can help. *Livelife365* can help.

I can help.

If you are still reading this introduction, I thank you. And if you are wondering right about now just who is this guy Mike Foster and why should you listen to him? I applaud you. Why? Because you shouldn't take advice about ways to improve and change your life from just anyone. You should have some idea who it is offering this advice, right? You are intrigued, aren't you? I mean, just a little bit, right? I thought so.

Turn the page…

WHO IS MIKE FOSTER?

(AND WHY YOU SHOULD LISTEN TO HIM)

Good question and one that anyone reading this book should be asking themselves. Let me start by listing all the things that I am not:

- a certified nutritionist
- a medical doctor
- a physical therapist
- a personal trainer
- a CPA, tax accountant, or professional financial expert
- a marriage/family/relationship councilor
- a psychologist
- a physiotherapist
- a dietitian
- a substance abuse expert
- a college graduate
- a professional comic, actor or performer
- a nutritionist
- a chef

Wow, that is one lengthy list of non-accomplishments, you should be very proud of yourself, Mike! Actually, I am quite proud of myself, but not because I am not a certified, professionally-trained degree-holder in any of the above mentioned very respectable professions. I'm proud because I feel that through a lifetime of learning from my mistakes, continuous autodidactic study, and trial and error, I can more that hold my own in any of those areas of expertise.

Q: How can that be?

A: By reading, failing, succeeding, recovering, doing, enduring, learning, laughing, crying, marrying, divorcing, loving, growing, sweating, eating, dieting, reading some more, studying, questioning, embracing, acting, singing, filming, being. Living.

I've given you a list of things I am not. In a moment, I will offer you a list of some of the things I've accomplished and learned during my more than half-century of living. But before I do that, here is another list—an accumulation of my failures. Why would I want to publish a list of failures? Because:

Failure = Feedback.

If you never try then you will never fail. If you never fail then you will never live.

Remember: **FAILURE IS A GOOD THING!**

Without failure you will never learn, grow, get better, stronger, happier, healthier. I am the man I am today as a direct result of having failed miserably from time to time. The key is learning from your mistakes, figuring out what went right and wrong, and then doing all that you can to make certain that that failure, or mistake, will not happen again.

What kind of failures am I talking about?

- two divorces
- personal bankruptcy
- excessive weight gain
- high blood pressure
- dangerous glucose and cholesterol levels
- heavy cigarette smoker
- long-time marijuana abuser
- alcoholic
- anger issues
- fear of public speaking
- low self-esteem
- depression
- college dropout
- job loss

No one in their right mind would publicly display a list of this nature unless they somehow overcame all of those items listed. Just as no one in their right mind would purchase a self-help book written by someone who is not qualified to help them.

The good news is I have overcome every failure on that list. And by using the programs and tools I've developed over the years to overcome these failures, I feel that, with my help, you can overcome your roadblocks and failures, too.

Of course, there's another option: listening to any one of the thousands of other self-help/personal guru/life coaches out there, the ones with all those letters after their names. Highly educated, doctored, certified, university and college graduates, with years of professional experience—why would you not listen to them? Another good question. Before you make up your mind about whom to listen to, I've got one more list (the last one—promise) for you to ponder.

My list of failures I've overcome:

- After suffering through two divorces, I finally figured out what I was doing wrong and how to improve my relationships. I am now happily married to the girl of my dreams, my soul-mate and best friend. We've been together for almost twenty years. Enjoying a lengthy, successful relationship is no accident; it takes a lot of effort, a self-discovery journey that I still have to work on all the time. I can help you avoid making the same mistakes I once did and better enjoy your relationships, and your life.
- Even after filing for bankruptcy protection after my second divorce, my credit rating and net worth suffered for years. But I hung in there, learned from those mistakes, developed successful financial planning, and now have outstanding credit and a net worth well in excess of the national average. Bankruptcy is not the end of the world, but if you continue to make the same mistakes and have no financial exemplar to offer his assistance it can be a huge mistake. That's where I come in—I can help.
- When you don't exercise, eat the wrong foods and too much of them, a funny thing happens: you get fat, out of shape, and suffer poor health. At one time I weighed close to 210 pounds, which on my frame is borderline obesity. But I changed my eating habits and created a diet that works (details of that diet and many other nutritional and fitness tips can be found on the following pages). The result: I lost over 40 pounds in only six months, and have kept it off for years. Losing weight and embracing a healthier lifestyle are major projects of mine; my goal is to help you see the same successes I have seen, and change your life for the better.
- While I was overweight, I also saw my blood pressure, cholesterol and glucose levels climb to dangerous levels. Through a series of

life changes and healthy programs I developed, I've since managed to reduce all of these vital signs back to normal levels, without taking prescription drugs—you can too.

- I used to be a cigarette smoker and smoked marijuana for years—just about every day. Believe it or not, quitting the pot was easier than the cigarettes, but I managed to do both. Overcoming addictions is something I understand and have been successful at. But it is not without its challenges, its fears and setbacks. The good news: I can assist if you're looking for help quitting yours.

- I started drinking alcohol as a teenager and during a long stretch of my life drank every day. I understand what it feels like to hit rock bottom, to let the booze take over, to have to consider drastic life changes before it gets too late. Through hard work and proper direction, I was able to change my ways, effectively changing my life, and can help you change yours.

- Growing up, at times I was unhappy, which led to my heavy drinking, which often led to being out of control, which ultimately grew into anger issues I needed to get a hold of. As the years went by my issues seemed to get worse. I had to do something, had to change my life. It took a lot of hard work and I made a bunch of mistakes along the way, but I finally figured it out…and can show you how I did it.

- I once took the same public speaking course in college four times before I had the nerve to attempt my first speech. I had such a fear of public speaking (a common fear, by the way, shared by many), that as a teenager, I broke down and wept the one opportunity I was given to speak in front of hundreds of people. I have since been an active member of Toastmasters, have acted in numerous theatrical productions, and have my own video website. That fear, and many others, is a thing of the past. Let me help you gain self-confidence and overcome your fears…whatever they may be.

- At one time I didn't think I would ever date a girl, let alone marry three of them. I couldn't interview for a job to save my life. And I used to get so nervous just talking to people at parties or other social activities that I'd opt to stay home rather than go out. Now my ego and self-esteem boarder on arrogance, depending on who you are asking. But it is better to be a tad overconfident than have none at all, isn't it? The first step is to believe in yourself, even if nobody else does. Over the next several pages, if you practice many of the methods and programs that have benefitted me, I truly believe that I can help you gain that self-confidence to change your life.

- Over the course of a few months during my mid-thirties, I suffered these life-changing events: divorce from my second wife, separation from my son, death of my father, bankruptcy, daily, excessive drinking, isolation, severe depression, overeating—I had nowhere to turn. I was at the nadir of my life, the lowest point possible, yet somehow I found it in me to dig out. I talked to some people, did a lot of reading and self-discovery, stopped drinking, started eating better and began exercising more. I took a road trip, driving from California to New England to visit my estranged son and morn my dead father. I went from a depressed, lost, broken man to a reborn, driven, changed, happy person. How did I manage? How did I survive? What did I do? Many of the drastic life-changing methods I used back then and still incorporate into my daily life today can be found in this book. My ability to reinvent and fix myself is one of the main motivations I have for writing this book. Why? Because I would love nothing better than to take all that I have learned and use it to help others who need help just like I once did (and still do, at times).
- Having squeaked by in high school, I somehow managed to get into college. Often distracted and not into it, I dropped out several times—one of my great regrets in life. But even had I graduated with a BA (I actually did eventually receive an Associate's Degree), I still would have needed to continue my education. Through a lifetime of book reading and collecting, a voracious appetite for knowledge, my desire to not just sit back and watch but to do, to lead, to help myself and others, to try things and fail and then learn from those failures, in many ways I have gained much more than most who've attended graduate school. With this lifetime of acquired knowledge, I've been able to achieve all of the above accomplishments, along with creating livelife365.com, a video website dedicated to healthy living, personal development, and entertainment. A website that has already helped hundreds of thousands of people change their lives for the better—an accomplishment that thrills me to no end.

Because of the tremendous feedback I've received from my website (and blog, livelife365.blogspot.com), and the countless people that have already been helped from my videos and blog posts, I was motivated to branch out and try to reach a larger audience. That's why I wrote this book. That's why on those nights when I am exhausted (after a day of full-time work and other tasks and chores) and don't have the energy to lift my fingers to my keyboard, dreaming of a warm bed and the television remote, I somehow make my way back to this workstation, to my websites, my videos, my vocation, my calling. Why? Because I have to. Because I am compelled to not only help as many people as humanly possible who may benefit from my knowledge, but to continue reading, failing, succeeding, recovering, doing, enduring, learning, laughing, crying, loving, growing, sweating, eating, dieting, reading some more, studying, questioning, embracing, acting, singing, filming…being. Living live every day in every way.

I invite you to join me on my continuing journey of self-improvement, a journey that begins, like all worthwhile endeavors, with one small step. My hope is that this book is your one small step that will lead you to a healthier, happier, longer, and more fulfilled life.

peace,

Mike

HEALTHY LIFESTYLE

I.   NUTRITION

CONSIDER THE ARTICHOKE

While cruising the produce aisle of your favorite grocery store, have you ever passed by a display of artichokes and spontaneously reached out and grabbed one? Do you remember what happened? Yikes, right? One of the

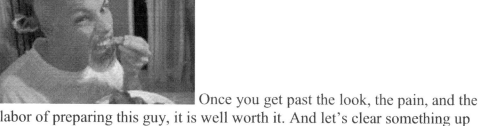

little thorns at the tips of this odd-looking vegetable   may (or may not—maybe it only wanted to attack me!) have pricked you. This more than likely caused you to toss the little bugger back onto the pile of like little buggers and search out a safer, friendlier veggie, like, say, a serene tomato or mundane carrot. And it's not just the fact that fondling (yes, I said fondle) this strange veggie may cause you harm, but look at the thing! It looks prehistoric! What with its fronds and thistle, its military green armor covering it. If you cross your eyes and look at it from afar, it could pass for a hand grenade. Eat it? I'm taking cover and running away from it!

But don't judge this book by its cover or this veggie by its thorny thistle. Once you get past the look, the pain, and the labor of preparing this guy, it is well worth it. And let's clear something up right now: This tasty treat is actually a flower. And the part of the artichoke that we eat is actually the plant's flower bud.

Being a Californian, this time of year I start to see fresh, California-grown artichokes displayed in the produce aisle. Peak picking times are from March through May. And speaking of California, here are some:

CALIFORNIA ARTICHOKE FACTS:

- Nearly 100% of all artichokes are commercially grown in the Golden State
- Approximately 75% of these are grown in Monterey County
- Artichoke is considered the "Official vegetable of Monterey"
- The heart of the industry is located in Castroville, who proclaim that they are the "artichoke center of the world!"

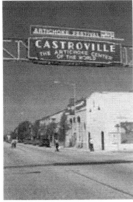

- (it says so right on the sign when you enter downtown)
- Every year the artichoke is celebrated with a huge festival in Castroville
- Cooler summers and frost-free winters of the California central coast, with the occasional fog keeping the air moist, are ideal growing conditions for artichokes

SOME MORE ARTICHOKE FUN FACTS YOU SHOULD KNOW:

- a member of the thistle group of the sunflower family
- if left to flower, the bud (the part that we see in the grocery) will blossom up to 7 inches and produce a pretty violet flower
- picked by hand and very labor-intensive using a special artichoke knife, a full basket carried by a field worker can weigh 80 pounds
- mentioned in literature as far back as 77 AD
- Spanish settlers brought artichokes to California in the 1600's
- Marilyn Monroe was once named Artichoke Queen in Castroville, back in 1948

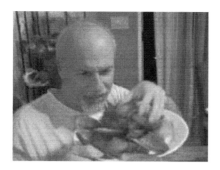

Besides tasting great, artichokes are high in fiber (6g) and have a decent amount of protein (4g). They are also low in calories (hold the butter!) and are a good source of potassium, vitamin C, folate, and magnesium. And speaking of butter…what is the best way to prepare them?

The most common way to eat an artichoke is to pull off the leaves and dip them into either butter or mayonnaise. I like to stay away from those fatty dairy dips and whipped up a tasty sauce made from spicy brown mustard, Dijon mustard, and olive oil. Try it, it may surprise you—and it's vegan-friendly. Which means it is nice to vegans.

I absolutely love marinated artichoke hearts, would eat them all day if I could, but don't because of the sodium. But I do add them to salads and sandwiches.

For some excellent artichoke recipes and for more information about artichokes, I suggest visiting these websites that I used for research for this post:

Castroville Artichoke Festival.org/Recipes

Gourmet Sleuth. com

Artichokes.org

I love artichokes. I try to incorporate them into my diet as often as I can. They are loaded with healthy fiber and vegetable protein, and they taste amazing. Okay, you may get pricked and have to put aside some time to prepare them, but they are well worth the effort.

The next time you're cruising your produce aisle, I hope you consider the artichoke. I know I'm going to.

peace,

Mike

I CANNOT TELL A LIE, CHERRIES ARE GOOD FOR YOU!

It seems I can't drive anywhere in town these days without passing a
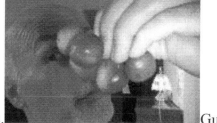
roadside stand selling cherries. Guess what?
That's a good thing. Besides all of these local entrepreneurs competing for
my patronage, the grocery stores are overflowing with these sweet (and
tart), delicious fruits. Living in California, and the fertile San Joaquin
Valley, I take it for granted that most of the time something fresh and tasty
and locally grown is going to be on sale. Right now…

IT'S CHERRIES!

My lovely wife is a major cherry aficionado, which simply means she digs
those chewy pitted babies. We can't drive past one of those aforementioned
stands without her begging for us to stop and grab a box. Me? I wasn't all
that into them until I met her, but eventually her enthusiasm, and that fresh,
juicy fruit, wore me down. Oh, and another thing:

CHERRIES ARE GOOD FOR YOU!

Actually, the more I researched the health and nutritional benefits of
cherries the more impressed I became. In fact, cherries are now considered
one of the **SUPER FOODS.**

Why are cherries SUPER?

- loaded with anthocyanin, a powerful antioxidant linked to their red
  color, many scientists believe a diet rich in cherries can reduce
  inflammation, lower bad cholesterol, and decrease belly fat

- they may help ease arthritis pain and gout
- one ounce of cherry juice contains the daily recommended amounts of antioxidants required to help fight cancer and heart disease
- cherries contain more anthocyanin (one of the strongest of the antioxidants, by the way) than raspberries, blackberries, strawberries, and blueberries
- one of the few food sources rich in melatonin, a natural body hormone that helps you sleep better and can reduce jet lag
- they help lower your body fat, thus help you lose weight
- can help control diabetes

Wow, after looking at that list only one word comes to mind: **SUPER!**

How do you like your cherries? My favorite way to eat them is the same way I enjoy almonds: by the handful. But unlike almonds, cherries are not nearly as fattening. One serving of cherries (one cup, with pits) has less than 100 calories (around 87), while offering up 3gs of fiber and zero fat or sodium. They are also a very good source of vitamin C and iron.

All this talk about super foods and health and nutritional benefits almost made me forget to mention:

CHERRIES ARE DELICIOUS!

Fresh-from-the-branch, pop-in-the-mouth delicious! Cherries can also be added to oatmeal, salads, desserts (cherry pie or cherries jubilee), as well as complimenting savory foods like pork and chicken. Serve them up anyway you like, but serve them up as often as possible.

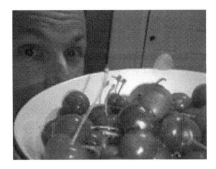

Cherries come in dozens of varieties, both sweet (Bing, Lambert, and Tartarian) and sour (Morello, Montmorency, and Early Richmond), in various shades of colors.

Like George Washington said, all those years ago when he chopped down that cherry tree, "I cannot tell a lie." Neither can I, so I can honestly say that I didn't realize how super cherries were until I did the research for this article.

The next time my lovely wife and I are driving around town and we pass by a cherry stand and she yells, *"Stop, cherries!"* I'm going to stop and pick up not one, but two baskets. Why? Because super foods like these don't grow on trees…uh, well, in this case they do, actually. I guess, what I'm trying to say is:

EAT CHERRIES, THEY'RE GOOD FOR YOU!

peace,

Mike

HEALTHY SNACKING THE FOSTER WAY

For the past few weeks my routines have changed as often as New England weather. My lovely wife and I recently moved from our house in the valley to a home in the foothills. While this move has been well worth the time and effort moves like these entail, the aftereffects are often discombobulating. Adding to the chaos, my main source of income—AKA: my day job—has also tossed some new wrinkles my way.

For the past decade, I have worked at home as a telecommuter. I have enjoyed the freedom and less pressurized working environment that

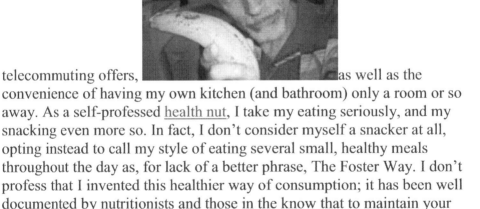

telecommuting offers, as well as the convenience of having my own kitchen (and bathroom) only a room or so away. As a self-professed health nut, I take my eating seriously, and my snacking even more so. In fact, I don't consider myself a snacker at all, opting instead to call my style of eating several small, healthy meals throughout the day as, for lack of a better phrase, The Foster Way. I don't profess that I invented this healthier way of consumption; it has been well documented by nutritionists and those in the know that to maintain your weight and encourage weight loss, it is better to eat several small meals throughout the day rather than three big ones.

But getting back to the recent changes in my life and habits. On top of moving and attempting to establish a new workplace, home, lifestyle, and routine, I now also find myself commuting into the office several days a week. This is not necessarily a bad thing, just another new change I need to embrace and deal with. The good news is I am actually enjoying this change in routines, but I have also noticed a few things while away from the comforts of home and my telecommuting life.

PEOPLE EAT! ALL DAY!

Now, again, that's not necessarily a bad thing if what they are eating is healthy. Remember The Foster Way. It's okay to eat every hour or so as long as the portions are small, you only eat until you start to feel full, and what you are eating is high in fiber and lots of other good stuff. Sadly, this if far from the case.

One of the motivating factors of my starting livelife365 was to share my weight loss and healthy lifestyle successes with as many people as possible. Why? Because I know the statistics, read the newspapers and websites, watch the news, and have seen firsthand that there is an epidemic of obesity and weight problems troubling this country and the world. Sitting amongst my working brethren, I can now add that excessive snacking is a major offender. But help is on the way!

FIVE WAYS TO HEALTHY SNACKING

1. EAT IT RAW

If you are going to snack, or graze all day, then instead of reaching for a handful of candy or another slice of that breakfast cake try a carrot stick or broccoli spear. Now I understand the desire to then dip that healthy sliver of veggie into some fattening dressing, like ranch, but try to resist. Instead, eat an apple. Or banana. Or orange or peach or nectarine or any of the dozens of nutritious raw options available. I usually brown bag a banana and apple and some cherries just about every day. Add to that some almonds or other nut choice, and you're well on your way to healthier snacking.

2. READ THE LABELS

If the snack you're choosing has more than a handful of ingredients listed on the packaging, then it's probably not good for you. If many of those ingredients are big words that are impossible to pronounce, then it is most definitely not a healthy option. Processed foods and snacks especially, are loaded with excessive amounts of sodium, saturated and trans fats, sugars and carbs, but more importantly, calories. Empty calories. If you are trying to lose weight, or just trying not to gain, then you need to limit your caloric intake. And if you find yourself in an office setting where you feel the urge to snack, then you will be battling a constant weight struggle if you consume empty calories: i.e. processed foods that have little nutritional value. The challenge is avoiding that giant bag of tortilla chips and salsa that one of your kind coworkers brought in to share, or those homemade brownies. Dive in and eat…but only if you want to gain unhealthy weight.

3. BRING YOUR OWN

What works for me is raiding my fridge and cupboard and brown-bagging it. When I am (forced to be) in the office, my reusable, recycled bag is never

far from reach. In it I have fresh fruit and other healthy snacks like soy protein bars or almonds or even a almond butter or peanut butter and jelly sandwich on whole grain bread (a surprisingly healthy food choice, by the way). While others munch on Sally's homemade breakfast cake throughout the day, I pop a few cherries into my mouth and keep right up with them, only guilt-free and happily healthy.

4. GET UP AND GO!

Exercise cures a lot of what ails you. When working in an office, or engaging in any other sedentary-like vocation, the opportunity to move around is sometimes limited. If not limited, the desire to move as little as possible versus getting that blood moving through you seems like the only option. I sit in front of a computer all day and often most of the night, but I get up and move around all the time. I try to get up at least 3-5 times an hour, if only to stretch my legs on a short jaunt to the kitchen for some green tea or almonds. I also take a walk just about every day, usually for at least thirty minutes. While at the office, I walk the perimeter of the building I work at during every break and lunch. Ten minutes here and there adds up—so do those calories burned. Remember: <u>burn more calories than you ingest</u> and you WILL LOSE WEIGHT!

5. JUST SAY NO

Nobody ever said you HAD to eat those brownies just because Sally stayed up half the previous night baking. In the perfect world, or at least the Foster World, all snacks would be good for you, and you could cram as many of them into your mouth as you wanted without suffering any adverse consequences. Alas, the Foster World does not exist (yet!), and constant consumption of unhealthy foods will cause all sorts of health problems. One solution is to replace that deli platter or nachos and salsa with something healthier—veggie platter, whole grain breads, vegan or low-calorie cookies, and fruit bowls. A huge bowl of <u>fresh cherries</u> is a delicious option to Sally's brownies any day.

Hey, I love to snack as much as the next person. As I stated earlier, I eat several small meals throughout the day, opting to consume my daily caloric intake this way rather than eating three larger meals with snacks in between. The thing that keeps me happy, healthy, in shape, and living life 365 is following <u>The Foster Way of Snacking</u>. You should to…but only if you want to lose weight and live a happier, healthier life.

peace,

Mike

SUNFLOWER POWER

Here's a riddle for you: What is colorful and happy and smiling at the sun when empty, but bloated and droopy and falling apart when full?

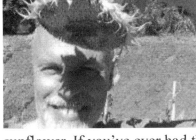

Give up? The answer, of course, is the sunflower. If you've ever had the pleasure of driving past a field of sunflowers when they are at their cheeriest, basking-in-the-sun splendor, you no doubt have witnessed them well before they are ripe and ready for harvest. Their flowery heads are tilted upward, soaking in the rays like coeds during Spring Break, full of color and promise. It is a sight I never tire of.

Yet when these stunning flowers are ready for plucking, they appear almost depressed: heads bowed by the weight of their plump seeds, once vivid yellow and orange petals now wilted and brown, leaves shriveled and battered by that same sun they once seemed to worship (like those aforementioned coeds, who right about now, after too much exposure to the sun, are just as shriveled and sun-battered).

The sunflower is one of those paradoxes I enjoy, a mystery of nature—a lovely flower that brings both pleasure and sustenance, beauty and, ahem,

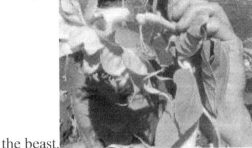

the beast.   For me, there is neither nothing as picturesque as a blooming sunflower field, nor as sad as one ready for harvest. But once they are beheaded (ouch!) and have had all of their seeds removed, they change from that ugly duckling into a swan of amazing health benefits and tasty treats.

Easy to grow and surprisingly easy to harvest, sunflowers are a popular choice for the weekend gardener—also a booming industry. Sunflower seeds are used to feed birds and baseball players; they are great in salads and in baked goods; and delicious as a snack or to start your day in your breakfast cereals. Sunflower oil is considered one of the healthier oils, high in monounsaturated fats and polyunsaturated fats, while low in saturated fats. It also has a higher smoke point which makes it a useful oil to fry with.

But wait, there's more!

There always is, Mike.

True, especially when it's about the healthy stuff.

Knew you'd get to that part eventually.

You know me well. Here goes:

TEN REASONS TO EAT SUNFLOWER SEEDS!

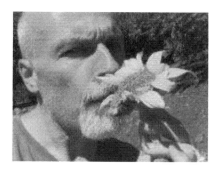

1. high in vegetable protein (around 5g per serving)
2. an excellent source of vitamin E
3. filled with good fats (low in sat fats!)
4. fiber! (Need I say more?)

5. lowers bad cholesterol (because of the phytosterols)
6. loaded with magnesium (which helps reduce asthma, control high blood pressure, strengthen bones)
7. fights cancer (due to the high content of selenium)
8. a heart-healthy snack (low in carbs and calories; high in good fats and fiber)
9. may make you smarter (from the choline, which helps with memory and cognitive functions)
10. **THEY TASTE GREAT!**

One of the staple foods for the Native Americans for over 5,000 years, sunflowers were a popular choice then and still are today.

The next time I pass by a field overflowing with sunflowers, either rich in color and basking in the sun or hunched over from the weight of their delicious seeds, I'll smile a smile of contentment and knowledge, while offering a silent homage to their amazing power.

peace,

Mike

PLUM CRAZY!

One of the things I love about this time of year is the bounty of garden-fresh fruits and veggies available. During my weekly visit to our local farmer's market, I can't seem to buy enough of the ripe tomatoes, crispy cucumbers, succulent squash and tangy peppers. And those are just the vegetables I'm trying to juggle in one arm while I ogle the assortment of just-picked fruit: apples (yes, the season has already started here), peaches, nectarines, and plums.

If there is a more colorful fruit than the plum I'd like to see it. Did you know that there are over a thousand varieties of plums in the world? With colors ranging from deep purple (insert favorite guitar solo here) and ink black, to bright oranges, vivid greens, and cheery yellows…name a color and, if you search hard enough, you will find a plum sporting that hue.

But I'm not crazy about plums just because they offer a rainbow of colors. No, I'm plum crazy because plums taste amazing and are good for you, too. Hey, you didn't think I'd be writing a about a fruit, even one as tasty and pretty as the plum, if it didn't offer nutritional benefits worthy of some of my past fruit and veggie articles:

Plums are part of the drupe family: fruits that have a hard stone pit surrounding their seeds. Other members of this tasty family: nectarines and peaches, two fruits, by the way, that I love as much as plums.

Loaded with phenols, which function as powerful antioxidants, plums offer a multitude of health benefits:

- a very good source of vitamin C
- better absorption of iron into the system
- reduction of bad cholesterol
- may fight some cancers, arthritis, asthma
- strengthens the immune system
- lowers the risk of vision loss related to age
- good source of fiber, vitamin A, B2, and potassium

Maybe the best benefit of all, when consuming plums in their dried form as prunes, is their amazing effectiveness in assisting with regularity. Simply put: if you're a tad bit backed up, have a heaping helping of prunes and your worries will soon be a thing of the past.

Quiz time!

Q: What do you get when you cross a plum with an apricot?

A: A pluot

Sweet and juicy or tart and chewy, plums (and pluots), along with all those other delicious members of the drupe family, are ripe and ready for picking right now. And the best part is they are low in calories and surprisingly healthy for you.

Maybe that's why I get a little plum crazy this time of year. You should too.

peace,

Mike

WHAT IS QUINOA?

A better question may be, What is one of the most complete (vegetable) proteins in the world? The answer is quinoa (pronounced: "keen-wah').

Last year when I was researching Super Foods, I inadvertently forget a few foods that several people pointed out to me were quite super in their own right. And I agree that there are dozens of foods that are just as super or more super than the foods I lauded in my video: ARE YOUR FOODS SUPER? One of those omitted super foods is quinoa. What exactly is quinoa?

Quinoa is often mistaken for a whole grain, but it is actually a seed from the goosefoot family. Today, it is mostly grown in South America, but it has been around for over 5,000 years. The Inca and Aztec civilizations were so fond of this super food they considered quinoa the "mother grain." Why is quinoa so highly regarded? One word:

PROTEIN!

Actually, two words: ***COMPLETE* PROTEIN!**

Why is this important? Amino acids. Most of you meat-eaters get plenty of amino acids as you gnaw away on your protein-rich meats; that's one of the major benefits one derives from animal protein consumption. It is also one of the main challenges for someone like myself, and hundreds of millions of others around the world, who has chosen a vegetarian lifestyle. Sure there are lots of wonderful vegetable protein choices, from nuts to beans to soy to whole grains, but few, if any, are considered complete, offering all nine essential amino acids. Quinoa is especially rich in lysine, which is helpful for tissue growth and repair.

Quinoa is delicious served on the side with veggies, or in salads or soups. It also is excellent added to cereals, and I use it to add complete vegetable protein to my Italian and Vegetable main dishes.

Why else should you add quinoa to your daily diet?

- excellent source of manganese (which helps with migraines)
- high in magnesium (good for cardiovascular health)
- fiber
- good source of iron and riboflavin
- low fat, low calorie food
- gluten free

Just because a food is considered super and good for you doesn't mean it can't taste good. I mean, I love broccoli and Brussels sprouts, but my wife tells me I'm stinking up the kitchen every time I prepare them. Quinoa is one of those special super foods that not only will help you live a healthier, happier, longer life, but will also add gastronomic pleasure along the way.

peace,

Mike

THAT'S AMORE!

There are few things in this world I love to eat more than Italian food. Okay, in the past I have admitted to a mild Mexican food addiction, and you know while on my frequent walks a handful of almonds are never far from reach. But when it comes to down-home comfort foods, my mouth salivates to the savory aroma of garlic and onions sautéing in olive oil, soon to be joined by crushed tomatoes, maybe some black olives or eggplant, all served over my favorite pasta. Makes me want to break out into song:

"When the moon hits your eye like a big pizza pie, that's amore!"

Hey, Dean Martin couldn't have put it any better himself. Amore means "love" in Italian, and who doesn't love pizza? Spaghetti? Ravioli? Meatballs? (I'll take mine veggie-style, thank you). And, of course, that all-time classic: lasagna! I was raised on tomato sauce and pasta, enjoyed one variation or another of it every week, but for special occasions there was nothing like my mom's lasagna. Whenever I visit my family Back East, the first question out of my mother's mouth is:

Mom: Michael, do you want me to make you anything special?

Mike: What do you think, Ma?

Mom: Huh?

Mike: You know.

Mom: Oh, yes…what?

Mike: Ma! Your lasagna! What else?

Mom: Oh, you like my lasagna, do you?

Mike: Come on, Ma, of course!

Mom: You sure?

Mike: Ma…

Mom: Huh?

Mike: Never mind…

Mom: I'll make two.

And she does. My mouth is watering at the thought. What do you have to say about that, huh, Dean?

"When the stars make you drool just like pasta fagioli, that's amore!"

Everything's amore with this guy. The real question you may be asking yourself is: What is pasta fagioli? This video may help:

Simply put, pasta fagioi means pasta and beans. And Italian comfort food that can be served as a soup or a main dish, it was originally created from the week's leftover tomato sauce, pasta, beans, and whatever else was hanging around the kitchen. Toss them in a pot, mix them together, ass some olive oil, fresh grated parm cheese, and you have yourself a mouthwatering meal. Bon Appetito!

Italian food, besides tasting delicious, can also be healthy for you. My pasta fagioli recipe is loaded with vegetable protein (24g) and is high in fiber (20g). And when you use low-sodium beans and tomatoes, olive oil and garlic, along with whole grain pasta, it can be a healthy meal option. Especially when you make your own marinara sauce.

Simple, fast and easy, marinara sauce takes a few minutes of sautéing onions and garlic, adding fresh chopped tomatoes, some spices, heaving on the oregano, and let simmer for a half-hour. The end result is pasta topping ten times better than what you get out of a jar.

All that's left to do is add some fresh grated Parmesan cheese and dig in. What's that? Dean has one last thing to say?

"Scuzza me, but you see, back in old Napoli, that's amore!"

No matter what language you say it in, I love Italian food! And when prepared right, it is not only one of the tastiest foods on earth, but also one of the healthiest.

peace,

Mike

WHAT IS PAPAYA?

Whenever I have the good fortune to visit the Hawaiian Islands, I take the opportunity to indulge in as many of the local delicacies as possible, be it

Maui Onions or locally grown avocados. There are few things I enjoy more than taking my morning walk, enjoying the always perfect weather, and checking out the farmer's market for produce that I don't normally eat here on the mainland

Many of you, I'm sure, have eaten papaya, have enjoyed its succulent flavor (like a peach, but different) in smoothies, juices, or diced in a tropical fruit salad. While some of you may have led a more conservative dietary lifestyle and never ventured deeper into the produce aisle to discover this amazing fruit, perhaps others are like me, needing a trip to a tropical paradise to awaken those salivary glands and indulge in diversity. Whatever category you fall under, papaya is not only delicious, but one of the most nutritious fruits in the world.

TEN THINGS YOU SHOULD KNOW ABOUT PAPAYA

1. picked while still hard and green (like the avocado), they turn pretty amber when ripe enough to eat

2. the seeds have a peppery taste and are often dried and ground up and

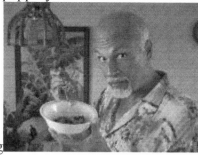

used as a seasoning

3. loaded with the enzyme papain: which aids in digestion, can tenderize meats, and even is used to treat cuts and burns

4. the leaves of the papaya tree can be eaten as a spinach-like vegetable and also dried and used to make tea

5. have more vitamin C than apples or oranges

6. Christopher Columbus called papaya the "fruit of the angels"

7. loaded with antioxidants, potassium, and folate, papayas are great for the immune system and may help fight cancer and heart disease

8. they have been used for both promoting fertility and preventing it, depending on what culture you consult

9. when eaten while drinking green tea, papaya may also help prevent prostate cancer

10. one of the healthiest low calorie/high fiber foods you can eat

I always feel like kicking myself whenever I get my hands on a papaya and cut one open, not because they are difficult to eat (they aren't), but because I realize, the second my taste buds scream with pleasure, that it's been too long since I last had one. But before I did the research for this post, I had no idea how foolish I'd been not to include papaya in my regular diet—they literally are, pound for pound, one of the best things you can eat because they are loaded with enzymes, extensive amounts of antioxidants, vitamins and minerals, and lycopene.

Here are a few ways to include more papaya into your diet:

- juices
- smoothies
- salads
- salsa
- served with fish
- jams and jellies
- curries
- stews
- or just raw

So, what is papaya?

A tasty, nutritious, versatile, and amazing fruit that you should make an effort to discover and add to your dietary regimen. I know I am going to.

peace,

Mike

IT'S A BIRD, IT'S A NAME, IT'S A…KIWI!

Hey, could be worse, I could have said "It's a Chinese Gooseberry!"

What am I talking about? Kiwifruit, or as it's more commonly known:

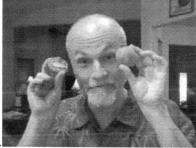

Kiwi. And, yes, it was once called the Chinese Gooseberry. Doesn't take an MBA to see why that name didn't stick around.

But isn't a kiwi a bird?

Yes.

And, isn't kiwi a nickname for New Zealanders?

Yes, again.

And isn't Kiwi the name of one of those new micro planets recently discovered in the galaxy Yerdaft?

Ahh, no, I made that one up.

But all the other stuff is true. There is a flightless bird in New Zealand called the kiwi. And New Zealanders are often called Kiwis.

All that Chinese Gooseberry stuff, you made that up too, right?

Ahh, no. That, I'm afraid, is true. In the 1950s, when New Zealand began to export kiwifruit, they changed the name from Chinese Gooseberry, for political reasons, opting to briefly call it melonette, and then settling on kiwifruit.

Besides having such an interesting past, kiwis are a delicious berry that can be used in fruit salads, desserts, smoothies and juices. As well as in many savory dishes.

But it's the kiwi's amazing health benefits that puts a smile on my face. Did you know that kiwi's:

- Are loaded with antioxidants
- Are high in fiber (eat the skin—it's fuzzy and tasty)
- Have as much vitamin C as an orange
- Have almost as much potassium as a banana

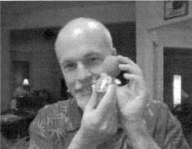

- Contain alpha-linolenic acid, an omega-3 fatty acid
- Are low in calories (around 50 a berry)
- Contain no fat
- Can help improve conditions of asthmatic children
- Are grown right here in Northern California (as well as Italy, China, and, of course, New Zealand)

I bet, besides wishing you had one of those juicy beauties in your hands right now, you're wondering how to eat one, right?

Easy—slice, scoop, or just bite into one like an apple, skin and all. Simple and delicious.

How do you know when kiwis are ripe? I compare checking for ripeness like you would an avocado. Gently press down on the fruit, if it's too firm, give it a few days. Kiwis are ripe and ready to eat when their outer flesh has some give to the pressure of your fingers, just like an avocado. And I know a little about avocados.

They may have a bit of a multiple personality and a somewhat sordid past, but once you get past all that, kiwis are not only sweet (with a little tartness, like strawberries) and versatile, but loaded with amazing health benefits—a good thing. I hope you enjoy a few today.

peace,

Mike

IN SEARCH OF VEGETABLE PROTEIN

I wasn't always a vegetarian. Back in the day, I used to be seated right beside some of you, gnawing away on that rib bone, masticating that filet mignon, devouring a double double from my (former) favorite burger place, In-n-Out. I was an animal-eating carnivore most of my life—just like over 90% of the population. Then I had some blood work done and got a glimpse of my cholesterol levels. Yikes!

Here's the thing: I was never what you would call a BIG meat eater. More often than not, I was just as interested in the vegetable and salad portion of my meal as the animal protein part. And once I'd done further research about the contributing factors of high cholesterol (mine, by the way, was closing in on 300) and unhealthy weight gain—namely: saturated fats—it made perfect sense to gradually cut down on the meats. Years before I became a full-time vegetarian, I often would go days without consuming any animal protein. My palette, as well as some deeper region of my subconscious, was changing, sounding an alarm: Reduce your saturated fats or die!

Okay, Mike, you can stop with the dramatics. But it was a wake-up call, and my unhealthy cholesterol and weight gain (I was up over 200 pounds—far too heavy for my barely 5' 11'' frame) forced me to do something else—discover healthier eating options. More to the point: I needed to reduced saturated fats, which meant limit the consumption of animal proteins. The answer:

VEGETABLE PROTEIN!

Here are some of the best sources of vegetable protein that I incorporate into my daily eating routine. Eat as much of this stuff as you can and you will not only get the necessary amount of protein into your diet, but tons of fiber (a good thing!). All without those harmful saturated fats; instead filling up with the good fats: monounsaturated and polyunsaturated fats.

NUTS

I eat nuts every day—mostly almonds, but all nuts have a decent amount of vegetable protein. In addition to almonds, eat walnuts, Brazil nuts, pistachios, even peanuts. They have anywhere from 6-8 grams of protein and 3.0 grams of fiber. I also suggest trying some of the butters. Almond butter is delicious and has 8.0 g of protein per serving.

BEANS

I love Mexican food, and eat it at least twice a week. I've found that you can replace just about any of the meat dishes with healthy black beans (7.0 g protein/7.0 g fiber) or refried beans (be sure to check if they are made with lard, in they are, opt out). There are dozens of varieties of beans: pinto, kidney, navy, garbanzo—add them to salads or eat as a side dish. Most have around 6-8 g of protein and about the same amounts of fiber.

And don't forget lentils. These tasty tidbits are loaded with vegetable protein—10.0 g. And 9.0 g of fiber.

WHOLE GRAINS

I eat a high-protein, whole grain cereal just about every other day. Kashi makes excellent products. Try their Go Lean. It has 13.0 g of protein per serving, also 10.0 g fiber. I mix mine with their Good Friends (5.0 g protein/12.0 g fiber) for a vegetarian protein and fiber blast (pun intended!) The days I don't eat whole grain cereals, I have some toasted whole grain bread (4-6 g protein; shop around and read labels, some have more protein than others. I recommend Milton's) with almond butter. You can see how the vegetable protein is adding up, huh?

Pastas, especially whole grain pastas, are another great source of vegetable protein. Most have at least 6-8 g, while some go as high as 12-15 g. Again, read labels, and you will be pleasantly surprised by all of the healthy vegetable protein options available to you.

I also eat oatmeal (8.0 g protein/ 6.0 g fiber) every day. And wild rice will get you around 5.0 g of vegetable protein per serving.

VEGETABLES

Not all veggies are created equal. Some have more protein than others. Here are the ones you should seek out when looking to increase your vegetable protein consumption:

SOY

I eat edamame, or soybeans, (11.0 g protein/ 6.0 g fiber) several times a week. I like to mix in another vegetable, usually broccoli (5.0 g protein/ 4.0 g fiber), add a little olive oil, salt, pepper. How's that for veggie protein? Also, soy chips are a wonderful source of protein: 6.0 gms--I like Glenny's and Gen soy. And Dr Soy makes a tasty soy bar (11 gms protein) that I devour most days.

ALSO:

Avocado: (4.0 g protein/8.0 g fiber)

Peas: (5.0 g protein/ 4.0 g fiber)

Corn: (4.5 g protein/3.0 g fiber)

Lima beans: (6.0 g protein/4.0 g fiber)

Brussels sprouts: (4.0 g protein/3.0 g fiber)

Artichoke hearts: (4.0 g protein/4.0 g fiber)

Asparagus: (4.0 g protein/3.0 g fiber)

This is by no means a complete list, and a lot of it is personal preference. But, as you can see, the variety of vegetable proteins available to you is endless. And the best part—they are low in saturated fats, high in good fats, loaded with fiber, vitamins, minerals, and nutrients that contribute to a longer, happier, skinnier, healthier life. Oh, and they taste amazing, too!

peace,

Mike

THE PASSION OF THE FRUIT

What is passion fruit? First off, it is one amazing, tasty fruit, but also one of the oddest looking. It also has one of the strangest names. Why is it called passion fruit? Spanish missionaries is South America thought the fruit resembled different religious symbols depicting the crucifixion and named it after the passion of the Christ: Passion fruit.

When did I first encounter this interesting fruit?

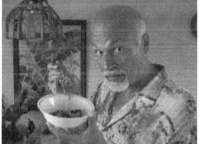It was at a farmer's market on Maui. I noticed these shriveled-looking orbs, kind of like a lime or lemon that was left out in the sun too long. The guy working behind the table grabbed one, sliced it open, scooped out its innards, and offered me a spoonful. I immediately recoiled at the sight of the gooey, slimy, seedy glob...and then he suggested I close my eyes and take a swallow. Man, was I glad I did.

If you have never tried this amazing fruit, you are missing out on one awesome taste sensation. A little tart, with some sweet mixed in; citrus and peach, pineapple...you just have to try it (and get over the seeds and slime) to really appreciate it.

But why else should you embrace this freaky fruit? Passion fruit are high in vitamin A, Potassium, and have a decent amount of fiber. They are also a good source of ascorbic acid (vitamin C). They even have some protein and iron.

Enjoy them in smoothies, juices and desserts, alongside savory dishes and in salads. But I like passion fruit right out of the shell.

Grown in most tropical regions, like Hawaii, passion fruit is a delicious treat, loaded with nutritional benefits, and versatile as a dessert, enhancing a beverage, or adding some zing to your favorite seafood or vegetarian dish.

One of the things I love to do while on vacation in exotic places is visit the local farmer's market. This is one of the best ways to taste the homegrown fruits and vegetables you may not have the opportunity to try elsewhere. While relaxing on the island of Maui, soaking in the sun and wandering through a farmer's market, I discovered passion fruit and still smile as I remember how amazing that slimy, seedy fruit tasted.

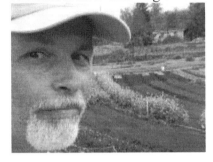

Ugly? Perhaps. Delicious? Undoubtedly. Good for you? Most certainly.

If you get the chance, try passion fruit. And always support your local farmer's market, you'll be glad you did.

peace,

Mike

FIGHT FAT WTH FIBER!

As much as I hate to admit it, I feel as if I've let myself go over the past few months. Okay, I know, I know: *relax, Mike, take it easy, Mike,; have a bowl of potato chips, Mike; that second helping of pasta is too tasty too pass up, Mike—LIVE A LITTLE, HUH?*

Problem is, I have been living more than a little these day. Having just returned from a wonderful vacation with my lovely wife, my belly is not what I'd like it to be. But more to the point, my overall health is not what I expect it to be. Now don't go rushing to conclusions: I am very healthy, nothing going on here that one would consider major, save for some weight gain. Only getting away from what I've made a habit of over the past several years, successful programs and practices that allow me to go through life with healthy cholesterol numbers, good blood pressure, and the ability to fit into a nice pair of jeans.

The good news? I know what needs to be done and how to do it. That's one of the main reasons I created livelife365—to share my knowledge and successes on how to eat right, lose weight, maintain a healthy, happy, lifestyle, every day in every way.

I may sound like a broken record, but for me, it all starts with fiber.

Alas, as the years go by our metabolisms slow, those cheating ways (see above videos) take their toll…and sometimes you have to slap those chips from your hands, and grab the almonds. Why almonds? They are loaded with fiber, have healthy fats, can lower your cholesterol, and are a wonderful alternative snack to, say, **POTATO CHIPS!!**

The key, though, is the fiber...and portion control. I mean, you can cram handfuls of healthy snacks, like almonds, into your maw all day and still gain a bunch of weight—there's no getting around the calories consumed

versus calories burned ratio.

But by adding fiber to the mix, your hunger pains decrease, because fiber stays in your system longer, thus taking more time to digest. Besides being full of nutrition, fiber also:

- aids in regularity
- alleviates constipation
- reduces the risk of heart disease
- regulates blood sugar
- provides energy, which helps you lose weight

Several years ago, I lost over forty pounds in six months. Since that time, I have gained some of that weight back. But any time I need to drop a few pounds, I always return to the program I used back then. What do I do?

1. Count my calories. Every day. I keep a dietary journal and keep track of everything—and I mean everything—that I put in my mouth
2. Make my calories count. I make sure I eat plenty of vegetable protein, lots of fruit and veggies, and maintain a balanced diet.
3. Limit my caloric intake. Depending on my weight loss goals, this can be 1500-2000 calories a day.
4. I work out often, walk daily, and strive to burn many more calories than I consume. Burn goals: 2500-3500 calories a day.
5. I do the math. The math is simple: you have to burn 3500 calories more than you consume to lose one pound.
6. I keep score. I weigh myself every morning at the same time. If you don't know where you stand then you will never get to where you need to be.
7. I load up on the fiber.

I also cut myself some slack, by taking the weekends, kind of, sort of, off. By that I mean, I will eat a slice of pizza for lunch on Saturday, but not overdo it so as to sabotage all that hard work I put in during the week.

And speaking of pizza—stay away from the carbs, especially the empty carbs (like those aforementioned chips). Since I am counting my calories and making them count, as well as limiting my intake of food, I have little left in my daily diet to add empty calories…unless I want to gain weight, rather than drop those excess pounds.

The other key is this: **SACRIFICE**!

You have to remember that that belly didn't happen overnight; it took months of pigging out and sitting on your duff watching bad TV. So dropping all that "Dancing with the Stars" weight will take time too.

My goal is the same it was when I lost all that weight the first time: Two Pounds a Week.

Lastly, here are a few of my favorite foods that taste great and help me stay fit and lose weight:

- Beans, lentils, wild rice, quinoa, soybeans
- Broccoli, artichokes, asparagus, spinach
- Tomatoes, cucumbers, carrots, cabbage
- Almonds, walnuts, pistachios, sunflower seeds
- Apples, bananas, oranges, kiwifruit, papaya
- Water, fruit juice, green tea
- Oatmeal, flax seed

Eating right is a daily activity—so is living a healthy, happy, long and fulfilling life. Sometimes snacks get in the way. The good news is you can always choose to change for the better

peace

Mike

WHAT IS JICAMA?

Many of you may already know what jicama is, may already know how to correctly pronounce it, and may have actually had some contact with it. If that's the case, congratulations on your acquired knowledge and worldliness—you are more than welcome to skip this next part.

For those of you still clueless—a pop quiz:

Jicama is:

a) a tropical island in the southwestern part of the Caribbean

b) a rare skin disease that turns the bottoms of your feet purple

c) a popular spicy stew prevalent in Portugal

d) an edible root, originally cultivated in South America

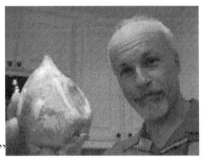

The correct answer is "d."

Jicama is a tasty, crispy, root vegetable, cultivated in South America for centuries. It is amazingly versatile, easy to prepare, and healthy for you.

Also known as the Mexican turnip or potato, jicama is used in many recipes south of the border. Its unique taste (a cross between an apple, potato, and water chestnut) and texture (crisp and smooth) make it one versatile veggie.

Enjoy jicama:

- raw, in sweet, fruit salads, or lettuce-based salads
- sliced or julienned to use with a dip
- plain, eaten as a snack (squeeze of lime, some hot sauce)
- diced and added to savory dishes: stews, soups, stir-fry
- mashed as a side dish

Once you taste jicama, you will ask yourself why you waited so long to try it. And more good news: it is loaded with fiber. One cup has about 6 grams of fiber, around 1 gram of protein, and contains less than 50 calories. Jicama is also an excellent source of Vitamin C and potassium.

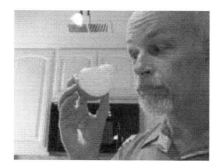

Simple to prepare, you peel jicama like a potato, using either a peeler or paring knife, removing the fibrous skin. From there, depending on how you want to eat it, it can be easily sliced, diced, julienned, or mashed.

Like my late discovery of the avocado, I did not taste my first jicama until I was well into my twenties, thus missing out on years of epicurean enjoyment. Don't let this happen to you.

The next time you're cruising the produce section of your grocery store, look for jicama, and grab a couple.

Jicama is not a rare skin disease that turns the bottom of your feel purple, but a versatile, nutritious, and fun vegetable that will delight you with its unique taste.

peace,

Mike

EGGPLANT, SO MISUNDERSTOOD

On those days (most days) when I am following my rigid, yet very effective, high-fiber diet, I often dream about eating other, tastier delicacies. You see, contrary to some popular opinion, I *am* a human being and *not* a robot conditioned and programmed for non-stop healthy living. Yes, I take pride in eating right, every day, as well as taking daily walks and engaging in all sorts of healthy activities. But, just like most of you, I, too, would love nothing better than to sink my teeth into decadence, often desiring to dump out my bowl of olive oil-laden veggies and nutritious salad and indulge in…what?

Well, as I mentioned earlier, I dream of my weekend "cheat treats" during those more challenging days of the regular week. And when I am not fantasizing about devouring a slab of my mom's lasagna, my mouth waters 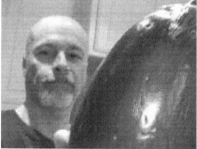 at the thought of another of my   favorite Italian gourmet delights: Eggplant Parmesan.

I love eggplant. As a vegetarian, I am always in search of great veggies to add to the haul that I consume daily. Prepared correctly, eggplant parm, and eggplant in general, will melt in your mouth and send your taste buds to gastronomical heaven. As I said, I love eggplant, but didn't always. Just the name connotes unsavory images.

Egg? Plant?

Yeech!

Like broccoli, mushrooms, onions, even olives, these were all foods, along with eggplant, that I refused to eat during my younger years. All foods, I might add, that I absolutely love now, as a somewhat-adult.

But eggplant? Is it a plant that grows eggs? Could that be possible? Who in their right mind would eat such an oddly named thing? Let's explore this often misunderstood vegetable.

Eggplants grow on vines, like tomatoes. They are spongy in texture and slightly bitter tasting.

Sound yummy? No? Read on.

While eggplant has been around for thousands of years, it wasn't always well liked by certain cultures. Because of its bitter taste, some thought it also had a bitter disposition: it was thought, at one time, to cause leprosy, cancer, and insanity. The good news is that has all changed. In fact, eggplant is loaded with phenolic compounds that function as antioxidants. Meaning that consumption of eggplant helps combat cancer, rather than causing it.

Eggplant is also a very good source of potassium and manganese, Vitamins B1 and B6, folate and magnesium. One cup also has 3 grams of fiber and 1 gram of protein. Besides those healthy antioxidants, regular consumption of eggplant has been found to help reduce bad cholesterol, fight heart disease, and improve cardiovascular health. Now all we need to do is find a few ways to eat it.

But first you need to buy a few. While eggplants come in many varieties,

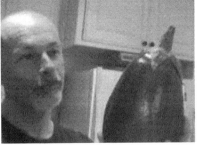 most of us are accustom to the fat purple variety that I am holding in my hand. To test for ripeness, gently press the skin and, if it is ripe, it should spring back. Store in a cool, but not too hot or too cold, place, and once you cut one open you should eat it soon--they perish fast. Now let's dig in!

Besides being an amazing veggie in my favorite (sorry, mom) Italian dish, eggplant also tastes great baked, stir-fried, stuffed, and used in another dish that I love to eat: baba ghanoush.

Huh?

Baba ghanoush is similar to hummus in that it is a Middle Eastern spread and dip made with eggplant rather than chic peas (garbanzo beans). I use soy crisps or strips of pita bread to dip into these two tasty treats. As a spread or eaten with sticks of veggies (carrots, celery, cucumbers), baba ghanoush is an excellent way to add eggplant to your diet.

If you have been avoiding eggplant, like I once did as kid, just because it sounds strange, or have yet to try it because your ancestors told you it may cause leprosy (believe me, it doesn't!), take my advice and give it a shot. If you love lasagna (and who doesn't?) then try eggplant Parmesan. And if you are in the mood to try something different, then dip a chip into a bowl of baba ghanoush. Or scoop out the center of an eggplant, load it up with just about anything, cover with breadcrumbs and some cheese, and pop it in the oven. You will be amazed at how tasty this misunderstood veggie can be.

peace,

Mike

ARE YOUR FOODS SUPER?

The other day, while reading the newspaper (and ignoring my computer), I made a discovery that made me smile, put the paper aside, boot up my laptop, grab a handful of walnuts, and write.

This is exciting news for me because I have been promoting healthy dietary choices at livelife365.com for years, foods that if eaten regularly can help prevent disease, maintain your weight, and prolong your life. Through a lifetime of trial and error, a voracious appetite for reading and the accumulation of knowledge, extensive research, and just what makes me feel good, I've discovered dozens of wonderful foods that have helped me lose weight, stay fit, reduce many illnesses and maladies, and, hopefully, will allow me to live a long, happy life. The cool thing is that many of the foods that I have long advocated and devoured on a regular basis have been labeled SUPER FOODS for their ability to do all of those aforementioned amazing things.

Here are some of the SUPER FOODS that I eat all the time, and that I encourage you to try to add to your eating regimen:

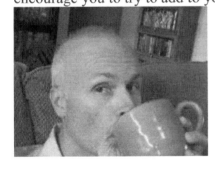

BEANS

BLUEBERRIES

BROCCOLI

OATS

SOY

SPINACH

GREEN TEA

TOMATOES

ORANGES

PUMPKIN

WALNUTS

YOGURT

WHOLE GRAINS

OLIVE OIL

FLAX SEED

QUINOA

ACAI BERRIES

CHERRIES

SALMON AND TURKEY are also considered **SUPER FOODS**, but are not on the list of foods I consume because I no longer eat animal protein— but that shouldn't stop you! Back in the day, when I was a meat-eater, I ate tons of turkey and fish.

Why are these foods considered so **SUPER**? One thing they all have in common is that they are **UNPROCESSED**. Most of them are loaded with

ANTIOXIDANTS and **ANTI-INFLAMATORIES**. Many of them are high in **FIBER** and **MONOUNSATURATED FATS** (the good kind!), and the best part: **THEY ALL TASTE GREAT!**

Many nutritional experts agree that a steady diet of these SUPER FOODS can:

- help reduce the risk of some cancers
- lower cholesterol
- manage hypertension
- lose weight and help maintain optimum weight
- reduce the risks of heart disease, stroke and diabetes
- enable you to live longer

The most encouraging thing I found while researching these **SUPER FOODS** was that the more digging I did, the more **SUPER FOODS** I discovered! And more often than not these foods satisfied my vegetarian lifestyle. Here are a few more **SUPER FOODS**:

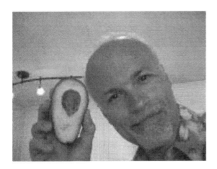

KALE
KIWI
LENTILS
ONIONS
AVOCADOS

BUTTERNUT SQUASH

The point of all this is not to hit you over the head with all these so-called **SUPER FOODS**, but to encourage you to try to add as many healthier eating choices as possible to your daily diet. Why? Because as I often like to say, *"Eat the right foods and the right amounts and you will enjoy a happier, healthier, longer life."*

peace,

Mike

I SMELL ASPARAGUS

What's the first thing that comes to mind when I mention asparagus? For me, it's not how much I enjoy those tasty green (or white) spears, though I can think of few other vegetables that I like as much as asparagus.

Does your mind automatically go through the long list of all the health benefits associated with a diet filled with asparagus? Probably not. The first thing that comes to my mind, besides the guilt associated with my inability to add adequate amounts of asparagus to my already veggie-loaded plate, is the, er, um, ahem…smell. That's right, the odor wafting up from the, ahh, you know, toilet…that aromatic red flag nudging my nostrils reminding me that, yes, I remember now, I had asparagus for dinner.

Could it be that funky stench is the reason why asparagus, while highly regarded in some cultures, is not as popular as it should be? Perhaps, like that pungent bulb of flavor, garlic, it is eschewed rather than embraced due to a particular lingering aftereffect of the somewhat smelly kind? Well, I'd like to change all that, melt away those stinky misconceptions and celebrate this wonderfully tasty and surprisingly nutritionally robust vegetable.

ASPARAGUS FUN FACTS YOU SHOULD KNOW (THAT DO NOT EMIT A FUNKY ODOR)

- asparagus is a member of the lily family
- plants are usually not harvested for the first three years

- after harvesting, the spears grow into ferns which produce red

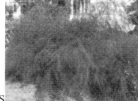

  berries
- a spear can grow up to ten inches in 24 hours
- the larger diameter spears are considered better quality
- California produces the most asparagus in the United States (over 70%)
- asparagus is one of the most nutritionally balanced veggies

Now, what about that smell? Do you know why your urine has a distinct odor after consuming asparagus? Before I get into that, let's look at the

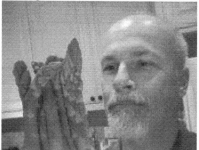

nutritional benefits of asparagus first.

A 5 OUNCE SERVING OF ASPARAGUS:

- is an excellent source of folacin (folic acid)
- is a good source of fiber and potassium
- is a significant source of thiamin and vitamin B6
- is rich in rutin (a bioflavonoid)
- has no fat or cholesterol
- is very low in calories

Every spring the asparagus is celebrated at a huge festival a few miles south of where I live. The Stockton Asparagus Festival is one of the most popular food fests on the west coast. While enjoying all things asparagus, you can munch on asparaburritos, asparagus salsa and nachos, and for dessert, asparaberry shortcake. Can you imagine what those port-a-johns smell like?

And speaking of that smell. First off, not all of us are affected (or afflicted) with that unique odor during urination after consuming asparagus, though I don't know too many people who are not. One theory has to do with enzymes and how the amino acids in this veggie breakdown.

I say ignore the smell and consume massive quantities of this delicious and nutrient-rich vegetable as often as possible. I know I'm going to.

peace,

Mike

FRUIT OR VEGGIE? WHATEVER, JUST EAT TOMATOES!

One of my favorite things I like to do this time of year is visit the local farmer's market and load up on my fresh fruits and vegetables for the week. This past Saturday, I was there—tasting apples and a variety of flavored nuts, while carefully selecting cucumbers, peppers, squash, and that market staple, tomatoes. Boy, do I love fresh summer tomatoes!

Recently, tomatoes have been getting a bad rap, with all the salmonella scares. And don't get me wrong—there are several crops infected with these serious bacteria. The good news: most of the tainted crops have been removed from the marketplace, and none have been traced back to any local area farms. I still suggest exercising caution (wash and rewash all of your produce, not just tomatoes), but do not stop eating these nutritious and tasty…um, vegetables? Fruits? Ah, let me get back to you on that.

To even suggest that tomatoes sold in your grocery store are of the same species as those bought fresh (some are picked that morning!) at your local farmer's market, is to compare eating frozen pizza to a fresh-from-the-oven slice from your favorite pizzeria. There is no comparison. Same with tomatoes. Store-bought tomatoes are months-old, stored and refrigerated for who-knows-how-long before being placed in the produce section.

My suggestion—Don't buy them!

My other suggestion—Grow your own!

My last suggestion—If you can't grow your own, then support your local farmer's market and load up on this wonderful…ahh, vegetable…I mean, fruit? Chew on that for a bit longer and I promise I will get back to you.

Why are tomatoes so good for you? Lycopene. This is the chemical that makes tomatoes red. A review of over 50 different studies showed consistently that the more tomatoes and tomato products people eat, the lower their risks of many different kinds of cancer. The evidence is stronger in the prostate, lung, and stomach. The tomato is also an excellent source of vitamin C (one medium tomato provides 40% of the RDA) and a good source of vitamin A (20% of the RDA).

Okay, well and good, Mike, but the summer-fresh tomato season is short, and you suggest we shy away from the grocery store tomatoes. What do we do for the other eight months?

Can it.

Beg your pardon?

The tomatoes. Can them.

Oh, I thought you meant…

Never mind that. For those months in between the too-short farm-fresh tomato season, I suggest, especially if you grow your own, to eat as many as you can, freeze some, and then can, or jar, the rest. You'll be pleasantly surprised how fresh and tasty they remain months after you have plucked them from the vine. As for the rest of you who don't grow your own—buy them canned. There are several excellent canned tomato products to choose from. I look for organic and watch the sodium levels. While these are not as tasty as the summer fresh fruit (veggie?), they still, in my opinion, are many times tastier that those sad excuses sitting forlornly in your grocer's produce section. And here's a bonus: processed tomatoes contain even more lycopene because the process helps release concentrated carotenoids. Even in ketchup!

What's your favorite tomato dish? Growing up in an Italian household, where my mother made a tomato sauce once a week, I love pasta. I could drink marinara sauce! (I'm kidding…I use an i.v. drip). But summertime, I love nothing better than slicing up a fresh tomato (still warm from sitting on a window sill to ripen. Do not put fresh tomatoes in the fridge—it reduces flavor and texture, turning them into clones of their pathetic cousins from the grocery store) and eating it between slices of lightly toasted bread, a touch of mayonnaise, maybe a slice of cheese, and salt and pepper. My mouth is watering. Hope yours is too.

So, what's the verdict?

Yeah, wow, tomatoes are good for you and taste great, especially in the summer. Gonna run out and—

No, not that. Fruit or vegetable?

Ummmm…

A: To really figure out if a tomato is a fruit or vegetable, you need to know what makes a fruit a fruit, and a vegetable a vegetable. The big question to ask is: does it have seeds?

If the answer is yes, then technically, you have a fruit. This means that tomatoes are a fruit. It also makes cucumbers, squash, green beans and walnuts fruits as well.

What does it all mean? Who knows? What I do know is this: call them what you want, but just go out there and eat summer-fresh tomatoes every day while they last. They taste great, and may just save your life.

peace,

Mike

WHY OATMEAL RULES!

The consumption of rolled oats is a common sight and occurrence in my household—I eat a bowl of oatmeal just about every single day. Why? Besides tasting pretty good, a daily helping of oatmeal may someday save your life.

It's true. Eating 3g of soluble fiber daily from oatmeal (about one small serving) may reduce the risk of heart disease, and can help lower LDL (that's the bad stuff) cholesterol. Chew on that next time you're considering bacon and eggs for breakfast—which, last I heard, is the antithesis of heart-healthy.

What actually is oatmeal? Oatmeal is rolled oats, which are made from oat groats, which come from oat grain and have been rolled to cook quickly and make them easier to eat. The oats have a thick bran layer that is removed through steaming to soften them. The end result is the oatmeal most of us eat. It is a whole grain that is loaded with fiber and protein. Now, if you omit the steaming process and just chop up the oat groats (leaving bits of the bran layer), what remains are steel-cut oats. You may have seen these in the grocery aisle alongside regular oatmeal. Steel-cut oatmeal has more fiber and protein than regular oatmeal—having never tried these, I cannot offer a comparison as to what type tastes better.

Besides being heart-healthy and a tasty way to help lower your bad cholesterol, oatmeal is also an excellent source of thiamine and iron, as well as niacin, riboflavin, folic acid, Vitamin A, and calcium. And if all those great nutritional benefits aren't enough, oatmeal possesses antioxidant compounds unique to oats called avenanthramides—these help reduce the risk of cardiovascular disease, as well as help lower LDL cholesterol.

As a vegetarian, I am always searching for vegetable protein sources—a serving of oatmeal has 8gs of protein, and that's a good thing!

Oatmeal also is an excellent source of fiber: 6gs. I can't think of many food choices better for you than whole grain fiber. Here are some of the amazing health benefits of a diet high in whole grains, like oatmeal:

• Lower the risk of type 2 diabetes

• Enhance immune response to infection

• Cardiovascular benefits for postmenopausal women

• Prevents heart failure

• Protection against breast cancer

All that's left for you to do now is eat some, every day. I eat mine pretty plain, with just a touch of fake sugar to sweeten it a bit. I also opt for the instant oatmeal—just boil water and pour, even easy for a simpleton like myself. You may also enjoy oatmeal with honey, chopped up bananas or peaches or apples and cinnamon. Blueberries, raspberries or blackberries also taste great with oatmeal, and increase the antioxidants!

Now do you see why Oatmeal Rules!

Is it any wonder why I eat a bowl of oatmeal just about every day? Is there any conceivable reason why you shouldn't do the same?

peace,

Mike

VIVA AVOCADO!

As much as I love eating avocados today, it's hard to imagine that I didn't taste my first one until I was well into my twenties. I grew up in a small town in a small New England state. Our foods of choice leaned more toward clam cakes and chowder than tacos and enchiladas. Avocado? I hadn't a clue what one was.

And don't even get me going about guacamole. Guaca...huh?

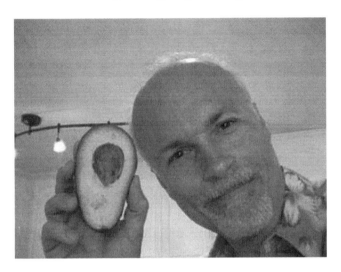

I understand that the avocado existed when I was growing up Back East, and they may even have been available at the local grocery store where my mother shopped. But mom never purchased one, never brought one of those green-skinned babies home. Believe it or not, I did not know *WHAT* an avocado *WAS* until I relocated to sunny California in the mid-80's. And even then, I wasn't sure what to do with one or how to eat it.

Today, avocados seem more popular and prevalent in everyday cuisine. In most restaurants you can find them chopped atop salads, sliced in between sandwiches, and, in its most popular form, as guacamole, that amazing green nacho-chip-dipping-taste-sensation.

While your mouth is watering, consider these interesting facts about the avocado:

- a member of the berry family, avocado is a fruit, not vegetable
- the Aztecs named it after the word, ahuacatl, which means "testicle," because of its shape
- they have been around since 900 A.D.
- they have been grown in North America since 1856
- also known as the alligator pear, Jamaicans call them pears

Most of you by now have tasted avocados, but if you are still leery like I was, back in the day, you should give them a try. You don't know what you are missing. But do you know the best way to cut one open? Carefully take a sharp knife and work it around the fruit, length-wise, pressing all the way into the flesh until you reach the pit. Twist until you have two halves—one with the pit; the other without. You can then either scoop the entire portion out with a spoon and then slice it. Or use a crisscross pattern, press the back of the skin until the tasty chunks of avocado start to literally pop off. Add some sea salt and pop in mouth.

To remove the pit: hold the avocado on its side and thwack a knife blade into the center of the pit, then gently rotate the knife around until the pit pops out.

Hey, next time you have that chip loaded with guac, happily remind yourself that besides enjoying a delicious snack, you are also getting:

- 10 grams of dietary fiber
- more potassium than one banana
- vitamins E and B
- 10 grams of the good fats (monounsaturated and polyunsaturated)

RED FLAG!

While very healthy for you, avocados are also high in calories and fats. The good news: these are the good fats--monounsaturated and polyunsaturated. These are heart-healthy fats and help lower LDL (bad cholesterol).

The bad news, for those counting calories or watching their weight, is that an average size avocado has around 300 calories--so tread carefully. I know that I can eat one all by myself, diced, with a sprinkle of sea salt.

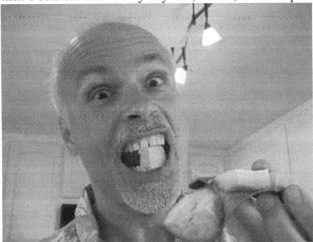

Try it! In moderation.

It's hard to imagine that I spent half my life deprived of the succulent taste of avocado. Maybe that's why I've spent the last twenty-five years eating more than my share, trying to make up for lost time.

You should too!

peace,

Mike

YOU DON'T KNOW BEANS...OR DO YOU?

I love beans!

Now there's a headline that makes one stop and look. Hey, I am not ashamed to admit that I am a bean freak, an eater of all varieties of beans: black, pinto, kidney, refried, garbanzo, lentils (which are legumes, part of the pea family), navy, and soy, lots of soy, or edamame. Why am I an unabashed lover of these colorful nuggets of protein, fiber, and taste? Well, besides protein, fiber, and taste, they are so good for you.

Beans are loaded with vitamins and minerals, like: calcium, magnesium, potassium, phosphorus, chlorine, sulfur and vitamin A. And don't forget antioxidants: the darker the bean the greater the antioxidants. Plus folate, which helps fight cancer and heart disease. Better yet, beans are a fantastic source of vegetarian protein (8-10 grams per serving), and for non-meat eaters like myself, they are just what the dietitian ordered. I eat one variety of bean or another at least once a day, be it while battling my Mexican food Jones (black beans and refried beans), or tossed in a salad (kidney, garbanzo, pinto), or as part of my nightly pile of vegetables, usually edamame. And I can't think of a better tasting meat substitute than lentils prepared just right.

Beans are also a wonderful source of fiber. And when I am not advocating the importance of beans in one's diet, I can often be found singing the praises of fiber. Lots of it. I eat well above the recommended daily allowance of fiber, which is 25-35 grams, depending on your size and caloric intake. Why? Because fiber is king: it lowers cholesterol, helps you lose weight by making you feel full longer, by digesting slower, and when it finally decides to digest, it promotes regularity. Beans are full of fiber. Depending on what kind you eat, around 5-8 grams a serving. What's not to love?

What else is great about beans and legumes? Fat. They are virtually free of fat, depending on the variety you choose. Read labels and be careful how you prepare them and beans will help you lose weight, stay fit, and live a healthier life. Also, when you have a choice, always choose organic. I have discovered some very healthy, tasty organic bean products that are canned. Check them out, read the labels, and you can find some healthy foods. Or buy a bag of dried beans and find someone who knows how to prepare them from scratch. This blog entry is all about the goodness of beans, not how to prepare them. By the way, if you find a good recipe on how to prepare them, let me know.

So, have you had your beans today? Try to make beans a part of your daily diet, like I do. You'll be glad you did.

peace,

Mike

AN APPLE A DAY

Sound familiar?

I recently wrote a post about my love of beans and their amazing health benefits. I received a lot of excellent feedback from vegetarians and meat-lovers alike. Encouraged by such kind words, I now will add apples to my long list of nutritious foods you should eat...daily!

I read recently that the average American eats about one apple a week. Now, given the poor and sometimes unhealthy, eating habits of most people, I was actually happily surprised by this statistic. But the article went on to state that for the maximum benefits of apple eating, you should eat at least one a DAY. Guess what? I do. I have been eating apples, daily, for so long I honestly cannot recall the last time I did not eat one. Wow, that's a lot of apples!

The good news is twofold: One, there are countless varieties of apples, from sweet to sour, crisp to soft, spicy to mellow. You have your red and golden delicious, granny smith, gala, Fuji, braeburn, honeycrisp, Macintosh, cameo, pacific rose, rome, jonagold, the list is endless, the myriad flavors countless.

Do you know that apples have been around for thousands of years? The apple tree is one of, if not the, earliest tree to be cultivated. Apples made their way to North America in the 1600s, and we have been eating them in this country ever since. Now about the second wonderful thing about apples: their amazing health benefits.

Apples have been linked to helping lower cholesterol, improve bowel function (one apple has around 5 grams of fiber, and you know how I feel about fiber!), reduce the risk of prostate cancer, stroke, diabetes and heart disease. There have also been studies that claim apples can improve lung health and help prevent strokes. One a day? I think I may have to up that to two a day!

As I mentioned earlier, apples are loaded with fiber, they also contain no fat, and have only around 100-120 calories. Besides vitamins A and C, you will also get some calcium, iron, and potassium from eating apples. Back to the fiber, one of my favorite health subjects. It is proven that eating a diet high in fiber will help you lose weight while maintaining a healthy weight, promote regularity, and help keep your stomach full longer, thus making you less hungry. What better way to increase that all-important fiber into your diet than with a tasty apple? A common suggestion for those trying to eat less and lose weight is to eat an apple an hour or so before a meal. Try it; you will be amazed at how effective it is in helping to limit caloric consumption.

In the wise words of Benjamin Franklin, "An apple a day keeps the doctor away." Sounds just about right.

Eat your apples, and all kinds of fruits and vegetables, load up on fiber, and you will not only keep the doctor away, you will live a healthy, happy, longer life.

Until next time.

peace,

Mike

BRAIN FOOD

I recently read an article about ways to stave off early dementia and Alzheimer's, and was thrilled to discover that I was practicing most of the methods already. All of the things I advocate at livelife365.com and this blog are great contributors in not only living longer, healthy, happy lives, but also quite helpful in ensuring that your mind is sharp and healthy for the duration. Here are some tips:

STAY ACTIVE

I am constantly going on about the importance of exercise, and there's a reason for it. It is so GOOD for you! One of the best things you can do now to help when you're older is start an exercise program. I recently wrote a post about walking that will help you get started. You will also benefit from lifting light weights (in the beginning) three times a week, and some form of cardiovascular exercise. Try riding a bike, either stationary or outside, treadmill, swimming, anything to get your heart rate up for 20-30 minutes, three days a week. As always, consult your medical professional before starting any new exercise program.

WORK YOUR MIND

We all use our brains in different ways, depending on what we need to accomplish. Most of that precious brain power is used to earn a living and maintain our households, relationships, or raise children. But to help keep dementia away, as well as improve your life now, you need to work your mind in other ways. Different ways than you work it during your normal routines. I do a crossword puzzle each day, which helps. Or try Sudoku or jigsaw puzzles. Anything that occupies your mind differently, works another part of the old gray matter, is beneficial. Reading is great for you. Toss out that TV and read, every day. Fiction, non-fiction, magazines, newspapers, ahh, blogs? Yes, those too. Expand your knowledge, learn new things--you will enhance your life now, and really help yourself as you age.

Pick up a hobby or learn a musical instrument. Join clubs. Do volunteer work. Challenge yourself and your mind and you will not be as challenged down the road.

DON'T SMOKE

Not much more I need to say about that except: DON'T EVER SMOKE! EVER!! There is absolutely nothing positive that can happen to you by smoking, so, please, don't.

MANAGE YOUR STRESS

First you take away my smokes, now you tell me to manage my stress? Jeez! We all have stress in our lives, there's no getting around it. It's everywhere these days. The key is finding ways to manage it. Here are a few suggestions: Yoga, meditation, long walks, breathing techniques, good relationships, making love (hopefully with the same person from that good relationship), laughter, and proper sleep. And proper diet (more on that soon).

I have videos at livelife365.com that talk about all of these methods.

DIET

Eating the proper foods and correct amounts of foods is something I talk and write about all the time. Why? Because I strongly feel that what we eat and their portions is the secret to life. Living healthy, happy lives now--and in our golden years. Diets rich in fiber, antioxidants, and anti-inflammatory foods will help you now and are being linked to helping keep Alzheimer's away.

Start with as many servings (at least 6, but 10-12 is better) of fruits and vegetables as you can humanly consume every day. The best way to accomplish this is to eliminate some other foods from your daily consumption. I have an idea--how about getting rid of saturated fats, unnecessary sugars and carbs, empty calories, and red meat? Replace them with: high-fiber foods like whole grains, beans and legumes, nuts, and those aforementioned fruits and veggies. And replace butter and other oils, whenever possible, with olive oil. It not only will help you age better, but it also reduces cholesterol and is loaded with healthy fats. Monounsaturated and polyunsaturated fats are the good fats. Saturated and trans fats are the ones to keep away from. Read labels and avoid fast food whenever you can.

And drink tea, preferably green. As well as rooibos and yerba matte. These teas not only taste wonderful, but are loaded with antioxidants, which help slow the aging process of cells, thus helping fight cancer--and Alzheimer's. I drink at least five cups a day--you should too.

Here is a video (Brain Food) about this post that may interest you. And most of this information can also be found in video form at my website, livelife365.com.

peace,

Mike

SOMETIMES YOU FEEL LIKE A NUT

Actually, most times I feel like a nut, in more ways than one. If you were to ask my wife, other family members, or any of my close acquaintances, most, if not all, would agree that I tend to conduct myself in a nutty fashion from time to time. Hey, I admit I can be a tad goofy, but that doesn't make me a bad person, does it? No, it just makes me a bit nutty.

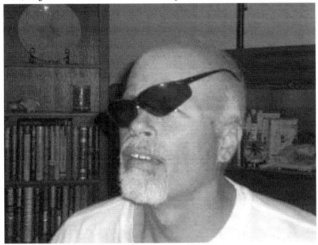

While this post isn't about me or my nuttiness, it *is* about nuts. I eat nuts just about every single day. And you should too. Why? Read on…

But first, here is a list of other titles I considered (and rejected) for this post:

1. Go Nutz!
2. The Power of the Peanut!
3. Almonds: The Perfect Snack
4. Ode to Pistachios
5. Wall-to-Wall Walnuts!
6. Have Nuts, Will Travel
7. Please Don't Eschew Cashews

Being a vegetarian, I am always in search of vegetable protein, and am delighted to report that nuts, besides offering us a (sometimes) salty taste treat, are high in protein. Consider these protein totals while munching your next handful of these popular nuts:

Almonds 8g
Peanuts 7g
Walnuts 6g
Pistachios 6g
Pecans 3g
Cashews 5g
Macadamia Nuts 3g
Brazil Nuts 4g

POP QUIZ!

Q: What is the most consumed nut in the world?

A: The peanut (Almonds are the most popular in America)

Okay, so nuts taste great and have lots of important vegetable protein, but why else should you grab a pile and start devouring them daily?

Fats.

Excuse me?

You heard right: Fats! The good fats, that is.

Most nuts are loaded with monounsaturated and polyunsaturated fats. Not only are these fats the antithesis of those evil saturated fats, but consuming massive quantities of them has also been known to:

  * reduce bad cholesterol and raise the good stuff
  * battle coronary heart disease
  * fight diabetes
  * improve bone health
  * help you lose and/or maintain your weight
  * prevent gallstones
  * give you more energy

Wow! No wonder I'm nuts about nuts! And I haven't even mentioned the fiber! Or the fact that most nuts are loaded with antioxidants, riboflavin, magnesium, copper, omega 3 fatty acids, and lots more.

POP QUIZ II!

Q: Which one of these nuts isn't a nut at all?

a. almond
b. peanut
c. walnut
d. cashew

A: the peanut is actually a member of the legume family.

Most of you know that I take a walk just about every day…oh, but the way, you should too! I walk so much I've even produced a video series called "Walking and Talking with Mike." On these daily walks, a handful of nuts are not far from reach. My nut of choice while walking are almonds, but don't hold me to that—I love them all! For those of you unfamiliar with my walking/talking/crunching routines, I've created this video for you:

SOMETIMES YOU FEEL LIKE A NUT

Speaking of almonds, I am lucky to live in one of the most prolific almond producing regions in the world, Chico, California, leading me to:

POP QUIZ III!

Q: What percentage of the world's almonds is produced in California?

a. 50
b. 32
c. 68
d. 80

A: c. 68%, with Northern California, led by Chico, producing the majority.

I love almonds so much, I produced this video over a year ago:

ALMONDS: THE PERFECT SNACK

Okay, class, let's recap, shall we? Eating just a handful of nuts is a good way to:

* add vegetable protein and fiber to your diet
* lower cholesterol
* control weight gain, fight heart disease and diabetes
* eat smart

And may I add: they are delicious!

Peanut butter is by far the most popular of the nut spreads. A dollop atop a slice of (whole wheat) bread, mingling with some (organic blueberry) jelly still makes one of the all-time favorite sandwiches enjoyed by human beings from age one to one hundred. But if you're only eating peanut butter, you're missing out. Cashews, walnuts, macadamia nuts all make amazing butters. My favorite, though, is almond butter. It has a distinct taste and is healthier than peanut butter. One of the places I love to visit right here in town is a locally owned shop called Maisie Janes. If you love almonds or are just looking for incredible (and tasty) gift ideas (their gift baskets are loaded with amazing products all locally grown in the area), I suggest visiting them online. You'll be glad you did. Oh, and tell them Mike at livelife365.com sent you.

One last thing: peanuts and, recently, pistachios, have been in the news lately for all the wrong reasons. Some crops of these healthy nuts were contaminated with salmonella, a very serious bacterial infection. I stress that you check labels and keep informed regarding product recalls to assure that the nuts you are purchasing and consuming are safe.

It's a shame that hundreds of thousands of people may deprive themselves of the enjoyment and health benefits derived from eating peanuts and pistachios because of human carelessness. My suggestion: Don't! *Do* play it safe and make sure that the next bag of nuts you buy is absolutely safe. And do yourself a favor and:

Eat Your Nuts!
(another considered and rejected post title)

peace,

Mike

HEALTHY LIFESTYLE

II.   FITNESS

TEN REASONS TO WALK EVERY DAY

1. INEXPENSIVE

All you need to get started is a good pair of walking shoes. Now I'm not
going to tell you these are cheap — good ones can run you more than $100.
But compared to the cost of other sports or joining a fitness club, this is
relatively affordable. You should also get a pair of sunglasses that provide
UV protection and have polarized lenses. Wear these not only while
walking but whenever you venture outdoors. No other equipment is needed,
except maybe a pedometer (about fifteen bucks). They count your steps and
can help motivate you to walk more. Other than that: socks, shorts, a shirt
— stuff you already have. And a hat to protect you from the sun. Oh, and
bring your cell phone just in case. You never know when you may need it.

2. EASY

We all learned how to walk a long time ago, unless there are some one-
year-olds reading my blog. All you need to do, after getting the proper
equipment, is properly stretch your legs (to avoid cramps or pulled muscles)
and choose a good route. Stretching is important. I stretch every day before
my two-mile walk and have, thus far (knock on wood), never had any leg
problems. If you're just starting to exercise or have some ailment, please
check with your doctor. Make sure you loosen up your hamstrings and
calves, ankles, and knees. For more on stretching, visit my website and
watch my video about walking. As for choosing a route, I like to take the
same route each day so I don't have to think about where I'm going. This
allows me to relax, let my mind run free, and enjoy the experience. Others
may want more diversity and opt to have several different routes. Just be
sure the route is safe, has plenty of shade, and is generally familiar.

3. VITAMIN D

There is a fine line between getting too much sun and not enough. While
you should always be aware and protective of melanoma by wearing a hat
and long sleeves, the right amount of sun, and the vitamin D that comes
with it, is vital to your wellbeing. The sun emits ultraviolet (UV) rays that

produce vitamin D. 10-15 minutes of exposure to the sun is sufficient time to get your daily dosage of vitamin D without risking overexposure and skin cancer. It is a paradoxical challenge, but one worth looking into. Don't take my word for it—ask your doctor, especially if you have sensitive skin or a history of skin cancer. But you do need vitamin D. Among its many benefits is improved bone density and lowering the risk of colon and breast cancer. Vitamin D deficiency has been associated with heart disease, cancer, depression, diabetes, hypertension, even obesity. So, walking is sounding better and better, isn't it?

4. SOCIABLE

Walking is one of the best social exercises, one where you can actually hold a conversation with your walking budding without gasping for air, like in an aerobics class. Some people enjoy walking in groups, and those can help inspire and motivate. Or just an after dinner stroll with your significant other offers significant benefits. Me, I walk all by myself, but I don't mind—I'm usually holding a video camera and talking to myself.

5. SPIRITUAL

Depending on where you are walking, and how serene or quiet it is, a nice walk can be good for the soul. My daily route takes me through winding paths with lots of trees and a scenic pond, away from traffic sounds—I tend to relax, commune with nature, and allow myself a time to reflect on things. Try it. If you are walking but remain uptight, you may need to rethink your route.

6. HEALTHY

It's about time I talked about the myriad health benefits of walking. You burn calories, exercise your legs and lower body. And if you take along a set of light dumbbells, you can even work your upper torso. Any form of exercise is good for you, but walking is easy on the body and still quite beneficial. Depending on your pace, you can get a decent cardio workout. And there's nothing wrong with breathing in good, clean air every day.

7. AGELESS

As I already mentioned, most of us have been walking since we were toddlers. And unless you are hampered by injury or illness, walking has no age barrier. From one to one hundred. Just be sure to select an easy route if you are out of shape or up there in age. But no matter how old you are, get out there and walk.

8. SAFE

As long as you stretch properly and avoid dangerous routes, walking is one of the safest forms of exercise there is. It is also, as previously mentioned, easy on the bones and muscles, compared to other forms of exercise—just make sure you buy a good pair of walking shoes. You can walk at your own pace, in a group, down a familiar path and improve your health and your life.

9. UNIVERSAL

You can walk anywhere, anytime, indoors or out. Using a treadmill or walking up and down the stairs inside your office building. Speaking of offices—you can walk around the building during your lunch break. The only thing stopping you is you. So, walk anywhere, anytime, anyplace.

10. FUN

Hey, walking is more fun that most exercises. And when you look at all of the healthy benefits I have shown you, it's also very good for you too. Get out and walk, every day, and you will be glad you did.

peace,

Mike

THE SECRETS OF FLOSSING

Habits often get a bad rap. Most of us, when someone mentions a habit, automatically think that they are talking about a *bad* habit. And, sadly, there are way too many bad habits that affect us in unhealthy ways. Smoking, excessive drinking, overeating, biting your fingernails, watching too much daytime TV talk shows, or even checking your blog stats every hour on the hour (I promise, I am working on it!). You get the picture.

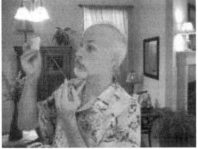

But I am also pleased to report that, while we all are challenged with the ongoing struggles to overcome our bad habits, a good many of us also practice *good* habits. I am all about good habits; like daily exercise, healthy eating, positive reaffirmation, personal accountability, and balancing one's life.

Psssst…want to know about a fast and easy habit that, when done correctly and daily, can add years to your life and save you money?

I'm talking about flossing.

For those of you visiting from another planet (Welcome!) or just recently rescued from a lifetime of living in the jungle or on a deserted island, flossing (from the ADA) " …removes food trapped between the teeth and removes the film of bacteria that forms there before it has a chance to harden into plaque. Toothbrush bristles alone cannot clean effectively between these tight spaces."

I floss my teeth every day. It's a good habit to get into. One of the many good habits that I encourage myself (and you) to practice to ensure long-term health benefits.

I am amazed by how many people that do not floss at all, let alone daily. And as the above video demonstrates, it only takes, literally, a minute out of your busy schedule.

Hey, calm down there, tiger! Why so adamant, huh?

Deep breath, Mike. Ahhh…okay, much better now.

Why am I so adamant about flossing your teeth every day?

Here are some of these amazing benefits of daily flossing, right from the dentist's mouth:

* helps remove debris and the plaque that collects between your teeth. This helps clean hard-to-reach tooth surfaces and reduces the likelihood of gum disease and tooth decay.
* makes your breath smell better
* polishes your teeth (when you don't floss, you only clean 60% of your teeth)
* may reduce the risk of diabetes, stroke, and heart attack
* saves you money, in the long run, by reducing medical and dental costs

I'm going to let you in on another little secret. For years, I did not floss my teeth. I'm not talking about skipping a few days here and there--I did not floss at all. And if that wasn't bad enough, I wasn't even going to the dentist for my regular checkups and cleanings. When I finally dragged my sorry self back into the dental hygienist's chair, I was given not only a painful and bloody reminder of tooth and gum neglect, but an educational lecture, spoken from the heart (my hygienist, by the way, is a very talented saint), that changed my life.

Since that day, I've now become a flossing freak, a tooth and gum advocate, and a regular visitor to the dentist's office.

Just like trying to do all that you can to find that thirty minutes each day to exercise, adding more fruit and veggies to your diet, or opting to pick up a book rather than the TV remote, dedicating *ONE MINUTE* of each day to flossing will enrich and change your life for the better.

Your dentist will be thrilled.
Your teeth and gums will be ecstatic.
And there's a very good chance that you will add a few happier, healthy years to your life.

Until next time…

peace,

Mike

BREAK A SWEAT EVERY DAY

To sweat or not to sweat? Sweating, at times, gets a bad rap, and when you think about it, actually ponder the merits of having your skin break out in a cold (or hot) sweat, it's a wonder we don't all go running for the hills. But there's the rub—if you did head for the hills at a good gait then chances are in no time you'd be drenched in sweat. But that's not necessarily a bad thing. In fact, sweating is as important for your health as proper diet, exercise, positive attitude, and the rest of all the good stuff I advocate at livelife365.com.

There are many reasons why we sweat—hot weather, exertion, sickness, nerves, anxiety—all sharing one commonality: we need to! Why? Because sweating regulates the body's internal temperature. When any of those above situations occur, you heat up inside. If you don't have a place for this increased heat to go, you're in trouble. But for most of us, the brain recognizes this warm up, sends a signal to the sweat glands, and, voila, in no time your hair becomes a matted mess, your armpits a river of sorrow, your back and belly, face and neck, hands and even feet are suddenly coated in liquid. Again: This is a good thing!

Sweating:

- cools down the body
- removes excessive heat
- regulates your internal temperature
- removes small amounts of waste (like chlorine)

But even more importantly, if you're sweating it usually means that you are moving around, exercising, working in the garden, playing with your kids, taking a walk or run, or just fooling around with your significant other. Many studies have shown that some of the healthiest cultures in the world find a way to sweat every day—you should too!

Is it possible to sweat too much? Or too little? Yes, and yes. Hyperhidrosis is excessive sweating, that, while maybe embarrassing or uncomfortable, is usually not a cause for alarm. But anhidrosis, which is a rare disease where one has little or no sweat, can lead to heat exhaustion or heat stroke because the lack of sweat limits the body's ability to cool itself down.

Pop quiz:

Q: Does sweat have an odor?

A: Believe it or not, sweat is odorless. It is the bacteria on one's skin that mixes with the sweat that causes body odor.

So, working out, running around, exercising and frolicking in the sun, getting a good sweat going is always a good thing, right? For the most part, yes, but you must stay hydrated or you could become very ill.

Symptoms of Dehydration:

- dry mouth
- tiredness
- excessive thirst
- weakness
- headache
- dizziness
- rapid heartbeat
- confusion

If you have any of those symptoms, you immediately should:

- seek shade
- drink water
- chill out, and drink more water

If left untreated, dehydration can cause a multitude of far worse maladies. Your best bet is to drink plenty of water while breaking that sweat and exercise common sense. Or, watch this video:

Breaking a sweat every day is one of the healthiest things you can do, just remember to replenish those liquids you are sweating out to keep dehydration at bay. And, as always, have fun while living life every day in every way.

peace,

Mike

LESS TALK, MORE ACTION

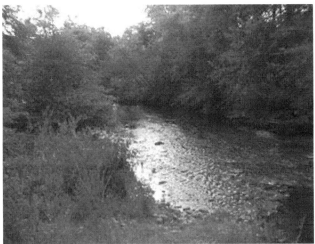

"Genius is one percent inspiration and ninety-nine percent perspiration."
Thomas Alva Edison

"Just Do it!" Nike

I don't know how many times someone has said to me, after I've told them that I have a blog and have written several books, that they always wanted to be a writer. I can only look at them, force a half-smile to my lips, and nod politely. What I would like to say to them is: "Then write." It's that simple. Blog entries, newspaper or magazine articles, college theses, and novels do not get written by talking about writing. As Edison said, you have to roll up your sleeves and get to work.

This blog post is not about writing, it is about doing, taking action. We cannot sit and wait for either the mood or muse to inspire us into action, be it while endeavoring creative paths, like writing or music or art, or any aspect of our lives. Often, I have heard others whine about not being inspired to do this or that. Again, I can only apply that half-smile and nod, thinking about that Edison quote. Because old Tom got it right. Yes, we have to have an idea, some direction, some clue what it is we want to do-write, sing, act, build a house, graduate from college, whatever-but sitting around thinking about it will never get the job done. Less talk. More action!

Take me and this blog entry. By now I imagine you have noticed that spectacular photo I have included at the top of this entry, and, no doubt, wondered what it has to do with all this talk about action and perspiration. That photo was taken at a place right here in town, a tranquil setting in the middle of our impressive park, where locals gather to run their dogs, bike, and walk. You see, earlier today, I was feeling sorry for myself. Why? Couldn't find that perspiration, or effort, to work. I was waiting for some inspiration too. Having neither, I powered-off this PC and headed for paradise.

The great thing about walking, while surrounded by lush foliage and the sound of water cutting through the green, is that it frees up the mind and soul, at least for me it does. I am lucky that my brain is filled with tons of ideas and thoughts crashing about, but sometimes I need to escape from myself, or at least this computer, and embrace the beauty staring me smack in the face. And while I was trekking through the meandering paths, in the midst of this Eden, I not only found my inspiration for this blog entry, but my motivation to write it. In fact, I was so invigorated that I had half a dozen blog posts figured out and found myself picking up my pace so I could get back home and jot them down.

What I did was rush home to grab my camera and click that photo at the top of this post. What do you think? Was it worth it? I think so, in more ways than one.

I guess the point of all this is that less talk and more action is good advice, just look at how successful Edison and Nike are. But more to the point, it is also nice to get back to nature, clear your head, and discover that once you do, you had most of it all figured out in the first place. You just needed to roll up those sleeves...

peace,

Mike

STRETCH YOUR LIFE

Before I take my daily walk, I do something that has helped me avoid injury, remain fit, and extend my lifetime warranty.

I STRETCH.

I perform a series of quick and simple stretching exercises that work all the muscles of my legs, from calf to hamstring .

STRETCH YOUR BODY

I have been on a steady exercise and walking program for decades and during that time I have not had one leg cramp or pulled muscle or any number of the injuries associated with the wear and tear of persistent pavement-pounding. Why? Because stretching works. Stretching warms up and loosens muscles and joints, better

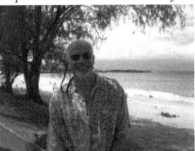

preparing you for the task at hand.

But don't stop with merely stretching your legs or other body parts. Stretch the rest of your **TRIAD** (*Mind, Body, Spirit*).

I've demonstrated several ways how to stretch the *BODY*, now let's:

STRETCH YOUR MIND

I often stress the importance of feeding your brain as much intelligent food (data) as possible. All too often, the mind is consuming too much junk food, or bad data. We all know what happens, physically, when you eat too much junk food: you gain weight, consuming too much sodium, cholesterol, saturated fats and sugars, which causes heart disease, diabetes, obesity, cancer, and other health problems.

Instead, stretch your mind, feeding it good, healthy foods (data):

* Read, every day ("A Book a Week is All I Ask"). Stretch your mind by reading diverse topics, explore your weak areas that need developing, spanning all genres, utilizing every media available: newspapers, magazines, novels, non-fiction, self-help, how-to, blogs, and websites.

* Learn a musical instrument or a foreign language. This exercises different parts of your brain, stretching you further.

* Continue your formal education. Full-time or part-time, go for that AA, or BA, or BS, or MBA, or PhD. This will not only stretch your mind, but it's also a valuable career asset.

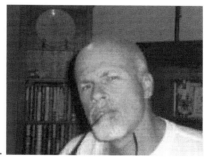

* Pursue your autodidactic education. An autodidact is a self-taught person, someone who continues his or her education through methods other than formal schooling. Never in history has there been more opportunity or information at your fingertips than today.

Stretch your mind, read every day, learn something new, explore the oceans of data available only a mouse-click away, while avoiding all the negative, unproductive junk food (data) that same mouse-click away. Your brain with benefit, just like your body, in the long run.

STRETCH YOUR SPIRIT

Spiritual fulfillment, or happiness, or just contentment, especially during challenging times like these, is as difficult to attain as it is essential in becoming he complete person we all strive to be.

If you possess great physical strengths and an exceptional intellect, yet remain unhappy, your Triad of Balance is lacking, incomplete. Besides feeling the pain of being out of balance, you are also spiritually bereft.

Stretch yourself spiritually:

* Give to charities, volunteer your time to worthy causes. By helping those less fortunate than yourself, you help yourself.

* Join local clubs or groups where you can interact with like-minded thinkers. Sharing thoughts, mingling, talking and laughing in a community setting go a long way toward improving your mental, happy health.

* Meditate, practice yoga. Relax the soul, and the body and mind will follow.

* Be positive, all the time. Easier said than done, but well worth the conscious effort.

*Perform random acts of kindness. Sometimes just a smile can make someone's day.

* Believe in the goodness in yourself, and the basic goodness in the world.

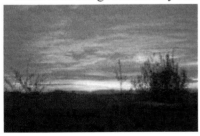

* Keep the faith.

Stretching is good for you. On those days when I do not feel like taking my walk or exercising, I still put on my shorts or sweats and slowly ease my body into my stretches…and soon I begin to feel the soothing, comfortable healthy ache that motivates me into action.

Make stretching your *Mind* and *Spirit* as much of an everyday activity as stretching your *Body*.

The benefits will far outweigh the effort.

peace,

Mike

HEALTHY LIFESTYLE

III.   WEIGHT LOSS

HOW TO FIGHT OBESITY

The numbers don't lie, the statistics are staggering, and the repercussions deadly. What am I talking about? In the United States alone:

- nearly 70% of Americans are overweight
- almost 4 out of 10 are considered obese

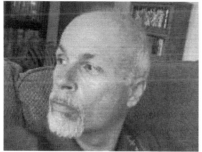

- 14% of children ages six to eleven are obese—think about that!
- being overweight shortens your life
- obesity is responsible for over 300,000 deaths each year
- between 1962 and 2000, the number of obese Americans grew from 13% to 31%

What is obesity?

From medterms.com:

"A person has traditionally been considered to be obese if they are more than 20 percent over their ideal weight. That ideal weight must take into account the person's height, age, sex, and build.

Obesity has been more precisely defined by the National Institutes of Health (the NIH) as a BMI (body mass index) of 30 and above. (A BMI of 30 is about 30 pounds overweight.)

The first thing we all need to do is find out what our idea weight is. This is something you should know, even if you are not trying to lose weight—given the stats, do yourself a favor and take a gander at these charts:

Ideal Body Weight Chart for Women

- Height/ Small/ Medium/ Large

- 4' 10" 102-111 109-121 118-131
- 4' 11" 103-113 111-123 120-134
- 5' 0" 104-115 113-126 122-137
- 5' 1" 106-118 115-129 125-140
- 5' 2" 108-121 118-132 128-143
- 5' 3" 111-124 121-135 131-147
- 5' 4" 114-127 124-138 134-151
- 5' 5" 117-130 127-141 137-155
- 5' 6" 120-133 130-144 140-159
- 5' 7" 123-136 133-147 143-163
- 5' 8" 126-139 136-150 146-167
- 5' 9" 129-142 139-153 149-170
- 5' 10" 132-145 142-156 152-173
- 5' 11" 135-148 145-159 155-176
- 6' 0" 138-151 148-162 158-179

- **Ideal Body Weight Chart for Men**

- Height/ Small/ Medium/ Large

- 5' 2" 128-134 131-141 138-150
- 5' 3" 130-136 133-143 140-153
- 5" 4" 132-138 135-145 142-156

- 5' 5" 134-140 137-148 144-160
- 5' 6" 136-142 139-151 146-164
- 5' 7" 138-145 142-154 149-168
- 5' 8" 140-148 145-157 152-172
- 5' 9" 142-151 148-160 155-176
- 5' 10" 144-154 151-163 158-180
- 5' 11" 146-157 154-166 161-184
- 6' 0" 149-160 157-170 164-188
- 6' 1" 152-164 160-174 168-192
- 6' 2" 155-168 164-178 172-197
- 6' 3" 158-172 167-182 176-202
- 6' 4" 162-176 171-187 181-207

I suggest you also check your BMI. Body Mass Index takes into consideration body fatness and size, giving you a more accurate idea of where you stand.

Now you have a starting point. If you're like most of America (and the world), you no doubt found your weight, for your height, on the above chart and wasn't pleased. Don't despair, this is a good thing. No, not being overweight or even obese, but at least taking that first step toward eventually getting you to your ideal weight on that chart.

The next step? Doing something about it!

One of my favorite mantras is: ***"Count your calories and make your calories count."*** By that I simply mean: if you are ever going to lose weight—and keep it off—you HAVE to, must, there's-just-no-getting-past this one thing: **BURN MORE CALORIES THAN YOU INGEST!**

The magic number is 3500. Why? Because it *IS* magic. It is the best way, from my years of experience, to lose weight. Oh, adding an exercise program to your life, eating more fiber, cutting back on fatty foods, and drinking green tea will also help you lose weight, but there is no getting around the cold, hard fact that:

"To lose one pound you must burn 3500 calories more than you ingest."

Getting back to the title of this post: Can we beat obesity? The answer to that questions is: Yes, but it will take lots of hard work, proper nutritional education, cooperation between school lunch programs and fast food restaurants, parents and friends, and most of all everyone taking personal accountability for their actions. Especially all you parents out there that have children who are overweight, obese, or bordering on either one of the two.

One of the motivations I had for creating livelife365 was to share my success in weight loss with as many people as possible. Believe it or not, at one time I weighed over 200 pounds, which one glance at that chart at the top of this post let me know that I was well overweight for my height and heading for obesity. I took action, and I am imploring and encouraging anyone reading this or who knows anyone who needs help to do the same— take action. Take that first step that will change your life for the better. I did, you can too.

peace,

Mike

3500—THE MAGIC NUMBER

At some time in each of our lives, most of us want, or need, to lose some weight. Whether it's dropping those last ten pounds that have been driving you nuts, or, like tens of millions overweight Americans, you need to drop a whole bunch. 20 pounds? 40? Over 50? Guess what? Do I have some great news for you!

If you can count, you can lose weight. Now, I know you've all probably heard a lot of this before—count calories, watch portion sizes, eat less, exercise more—but not all weight reduction programs are created equal. Still overweight? Still need some help? Read on…

3500

That's the magic number of calories that makes up one pound of weight loss.

Huh?

Okay, I understand, no one said there was going to be math, right?

Let's say you eat 2000 calories each day (which, depending on your body size, gender, or age, is a nice, average number to go by). Now multiply that by 7 days, and the result is that you will consume 14,000 calories per week. Here's where that magic number—**3500**—comes into play.

If your goal is to lose one pound a week, you will need to burn **3500** calories **more** than you ingest, per week. Using the above example: if you consume 14,000 calories, you would need to burn 17,500 to lose one pound in a week. Now, take those 17,500 calories and divide by 7 (days). That's 2500. That's how many calories you would need to burn, on average, per day, to lose one pound.

Wow, sounds like a lot of math, and hard work.

Actually, it's a lot easier than you could imagine.

Using this formula, and eating a high-fiber, low-fat diet, I lost over 40 pounds in only six months. And I have been able to keep all of the weight off for over two years. And here's the best news—burning calories is not that difficult. We burn them while asleep! You are burning some right now just reading this post. I burned a bunch writing it!

One of the best ways to burn more calories, though, is to become more active. You don't have to go crazy and start training for an Iron Man competition, you just need to get up and get going. Start a walking program, work in the yard landscaping or gardening, use the stairs instead of the elevator, clean the house (yup, burns lots of calories). Even going grocery shopping will burn a bunch. The Internet is loaded with counters that will help you keep track of all the calories you burn. The good news—burning 2500-3000 calories (or more!) per day is not that difficult to do. The challenge for most of us is consuming fewer calories. That's why I titled this post: Make Your Calories Count.

If you are to limit caloric consumption (eat less), then you need to make sure everything you put in your mouth has value and nutritional purpose. This means—no empty calories. An empty calorie is something (a bag of chips, slice of cake, most fast foods) that fills your stomach, but gives little in return—no nutrition, few vitamins or minerals. They may even be high in saturated fats, sodium, and sugar. No value—don't eat them.

Here's the important thing to understand—if you seriously want to lose weight and decide to limit your caloric intake, you need to ensure that every calorie you consume has a purpose. Why? Because you only have so many in each day/week, to waste any could lead to your weight loss downfall. An example: one trip through that drive-thru window at your favorite (not anymore, I hope) burger joint could blow your calorie count for the entire day. A double cheeseburger, large fry, and soda or shake, depending on which grease house you are visiting, have anywhere from 1000-2000 calories. And watch their salads; most are high in sodium and calories. My advice: Don't go there!

If you are serious about dropping those last ten pounds or ready to take that first step toward losing fifty, or more, count your calories (**magic number: 3500**), and make your calories count.

Here are a few more tips that have helped me:

- Eat small mini-meals throughout the day, every 2-3 hours. Toss out the traditional thinking that you need to eat breakfast, lunch, and dinner.
- Chew gum in between meals. You'd be amazed at how effective this it.
- Eat lots of fiber and less animal protein. Fiber curbs your appetite, digests slowly, helps with regularity, and is good for you.
- Stop eating **before** you feel full. It can take ten minutes or more before the brain realizes that the stomach is full. We all too often continue to eat way longer than we need to.
- Keep a journal. Jot down everything you eat each day— and I mean everything! This includes "tastes" while cooking and "nibbles" from your kid's or spouses' plates. And don't forget liquids; they count too. This is an excellent way to monitor what is working or not in your diet. I still have my journals!
- Walk. Walking is the easiest, least expensive exercise there is.

Remember—**3500** calories equals one pound. Burn more than **3500** calories than you ingest and you will lose a pound of weight. Do this every week and, before you know it, you will be well on your way to a healthier, happier, better life. I hope these tips help.

peace,

Mike

THE KEY TO LOSING WEIGHT

These days, just about everyone needs to drop a few excess pounds; for some, even more than a few. But let's face it, losing weight is difficult, and keeping it off is sometimes even more of a challenge.

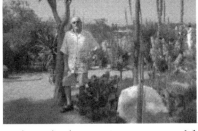Hey, if losing weight and getting into swimsuit shape was easy, we'd all look like models and movie stars. Sadly, this is far from the case.

But there is good news for those of us (yes, me too; I am constantly working on my weight. Even though I am at a very healthy weight right now, I know that if I didn't work at it I would be overweight and unhealthy very fast) looking to lose weight and keep it off; help is on the way. The key is to **COUNT YOUR CALORIES AND MAKE YOUR CALORIES COUNT!**

Sounds simple enough, and it is in theory. So then why are six out of ten people overweight? And over 30%, and growing at an alarming rate, considered obese? As I stated earlier, if it was easy to lose weight, we'd all look like Brad and Angelina. But we don't and it's not, but there is hope. Read on…

Any successful weight loss program, be it Weight Watchers or Atkins or Slim Fast or South Beach (the list goes on and on, doesn't it?), has one thing in common: you must burn more calories than you consume to lose weight. There is no getting around this; it is a proven and steadfast fact.

TO LOSE ONE POUND YOU MUST BURN 3500 CALORIES MORE THAN YOU CONSUME!

3500. That is the magic number. In this day and age, people are looking for a magic pill, something to pop in their mouths to make all of their problems, like being overweight, go away. Here's a scoop for you: **THERE IS NO MAGIC PILL!**

But there is magic!

- Magic foods! Foods rich in fiber (like fruits, nuts, whole grains, beans, soy, vegetables) are not only extremely healthy for you (most are loaded with antioxidants, tons of vitamins and nutritious minerals that help combat heart disease, cancer, diabetes, gastrointestinal maladies, and lots more), but WILL help you lose weight. Why? They remain in your stomach and digestive system longer, helping you to feel full longer, thus keeping you away from snacking and overeating. Fiber also promotes regularity and is a

natural colon cleanser.

- Magic numbers, like: 3500. As I previous mentioned, the only way to lose weight is to burn more calories than you ingest. And the only way to lose a pound is to burn 3500 calories more than you ingest. It's that easy; the math at least is. The rest is up to you. Here's a simple suggestion: set daily caloric goals. An example: limit yourself to consuming 2000 calories a day. Then set a goal to burn at least 2500 calories each day. That will give you 500 net calories burned each day. Multiply that 500 x 7 days, and you have 3500. Using this formula you are guaranteed to lose at least one pound per week. Could it really be that easy?

YES!…and no. Because if it were that easy…ah, you know the rest.

But it can be done, and if you put your mind to it, are sufficiently motivated and really want to lose weight, as well as being ready to change your life, then it is that simple…you just gotta do it! And I'm here to help.

Let's go back to my key to losing weight: <u>**COUNT YOUR CALORIES AND MAKE YOUR CALORIES COUNT!**</u>

The first thing you need to do, literally, is to start counting. Everything that goes near your mouth, including: tasting while cooking, finishing a few bites from your kid's plate, any and all beverages, all snacking and any sneaking. Remember, you want and need to lose weight, right? Then you're only kidding yourself if you sneak a few bites here or there…right?

Back to the counting. Get yourself a nutritional book that lists content of all food that you think you will ever consume. I like this one: <u>The Complete Book of Food Counts</u>. Also, the Internet has several excellent sites that

offer calorie counters for free. A few tips: dining out every night will make this task that much more difficult. Why? Because you will have a tough time estimating the caloric content of what's on your plate at your local diner, thus making it that much more of a challenge to count your calories. My solution: make your own during the workweek, and then, maybe, treat yourself to a nice dinner or two on the weekend. In fact, I encourage you to cut yourself a little break on the weekend, especially if you had a good week of calorie counting and weight loss. Ya gotta live, too, right?

Okay, so you have a goal of 2000 calories per day and you have been counting EVERYTHING that you've been consuming. I bet you're finding it difficult to stay within that 2000 calorie threshold, right? Believe me, I feel your pain. This is where the "make your calories count" part comes into play. It is essential to make each calorie you consume count while on a limited caloric diet. Why? Because you need to eat a balanced diet of fruits and veggies, carbs and proteins, fats (yes, fats! The good fats, that is) and dairy. And if you're limiting yourself to only 2000 calories, those will add up quickly. The key, again, is:

COUNT YOUR CALORIES AND MAKE YOUR CALORIES COUNT!

This is why keeping a journal of everything you consume daily is important. Write it down and keep score, making sure that you not only watch how much you're consuming, but WHAT you are consuming. The sad fact is you could eat a diet of nothing but potato chips, limiting yourself to only 2000 calories, and if you burn over 2500 calories a day, you WILL lose weight. But you won't be doing it in a healthy way. And why is this a bad thing? Your body will rebel; you will be unhealthy, tired, vitamin, mineral, and nutrient deprived, and eventually breakdown. So, again, the key (for those of you who have not been paying attention) is to:

COUNT YOUR CALORIES AND MAKE YOUR CALORIES COUNT!

When *I lost all my weight*, I kept a daily journal, listing EVERYTHING I ate. I also loaded up my plate with fiber-rich foods. Here is a typical day:

Apple

Banana

Oatmeal

Soy bar

Almonds

Orange or peach

Soy chips (snack) with hummus

Either almond butter or peanut butter on whole grain bread, or a high fiber and high protein whole grain cereal with soy milk

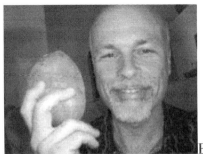Baked potato (no butter, just a splash of olive oil)

Mix of veggies: broccoli, soy, beans, carrots, cauliflower, etc.

Large salad (lettuce, cabbage, tomatoes, cukes, with some type of bean: garbanzo, kidney, black). Low-cal, no-fat dressing

Believe it or not, all that food rarely exceeded 2000 calories. Notice there is no animal protein on my list, but feel free to add fish or poultry to yours. Just make sure you limit your caloric intake. I choose a vegetarian lifestyle for many reasons, improved health being a major factor, but the lower caloric intake and extra fiber are equally beneficial.

I'm not suggesting you become a vegetarian; I'm just giving you a glimpse of what worked for me. Your list may be far different than mine, and that's okay, as long as you count your calories and eat a complete, well balanced diet.

Remember, if you are reading this then you are probably interested in discovering new ways of losing weight. My way, my key, worked, and continues to work, for me. I know it will work for you too. But you have to be ready, willing, and committed to doing what it takes to be what you want to be. Hey, what have you got to lose…except all those excess pounds. Good luck, I'm pulling for you.

peace,

Mike

ON DIET, NUTRITION, AND WEIGHT LOSS

As much as I hate to admit it, I feel as if I've let myself go over the past few months. Okay, I know, I know: *relax, Mike, take it easy, Mike,; have a bowl of potato chips, Mike; that second helping of pasta is too tasty too pass up, Mike—LIVE A LITTLE, HUH?*

Problem is, I have been living more than a little these day. Having just returned from a wonderful vacation with my lovely wife, my belly is not what I'd like it to be. But more to the point, my overall health is not what I expect it to be. Now don't go rushing to conclusions: I am very healthy, nothing going on here that one would consider major, save for some weight gain. Only getting away from what I've made a habit of over the past several years, successful programs and practices that allow me to go through life with healthy cholesterol numbers, good blood pressure, and the ability to fit into a nice pair of jeans.

The good news? I know what needs to be done and how to do it. That's one of the main reasons I created this blog and my video site, livelife365.com—to share my knowledge and successes on how to eat right, lose weight, maintain a healthy, happy, lifestyle, every day in every way.

I may sound like a broken record, but for me, it all starts with fiber.

Alas, as the years go by our metabolisms slow, those cheating ways (see above videos) take their toll…and sometimes you have to slap those chips from your hands, and grab the almonds. Why almonds? They are loaded with fiber, have healthy fats, can lower your cholesterol, and are a wonderful alternative snack to, say, **POTATO CHIPS!!**

The key, though, is the fiber…and portion control. I mean, you can cram handfuls of healthy snacks, like almonds, into your maw all day and still gain a bunch of weight—there's no getting around the calories consumed versus calories burned ration.

But by adding fiber to the mix, your hunger pains decrease, because fiber stays in your system longer, thus taking more time to digest. Besides being full of nutrition, fiber also:

· aids in regularity

· alleviates constipation

· reduces the risk of heart disease

· regulates blood sugar

· provides energy, which helps you lose weight

Several years ago, I lost over forty pounds in six months. Since that time, I have gained some of that weight back. But any time I need to drop a few pounds, I always return to the program I used back then. What do I do?

1. Count my calories. Every day. I keep a dietary journal and keep track of everything—and I mean everything—that I put in my mouth

2. Make my calories count. I make sure I eat plenty of vegetable protein, lots of fruit and veggies, and maintain a balanced diet.

3. Limit my caloric intake. Depending on my weight loss goals, this can be 1500-2000 calories a day.

4. I workout often, walk daily, and strive to burn many more calories than I consume. Burn goals: 2500-3500 calories a day.

5. I do the math. The math is simple: you have to burn 3500 calories

more than you consume to lose one pound.

6. I keep score. I weigh myself every morning at the same time. If you don't know where you stand then you will never get to where you need to be.

7. I load up on the fiber (see above and this video)…

I also cut myself some slack, by taking the weekends, kind of, sort of, off. By that I mean, I will eat a slice of pizza for lunch on Saturday, but not overdo it so as to sabotage all that hard work I put in during the week.

And speaking of pizza—stay away from the carbs, especially the empty carbs (like those aforementioned chips). Since I am counting my calories and making them count, as well as limiting my intake of food, I have little left in my dietary regiment to add empty calories to my diet…unless I want to gain weight, rather than drop those excess pounds.

The other key is this: **SACRIFICE**!

You have to remember that that belly didn't happen overnight; it took months of pigging out and sitting on your duff watching bad TV. So dropping all that "Dancing With The Stars" weight will take time too.

My goal is the same it was when I lost all that weight the first time: Two Pounds a Week.

And lastly, here are a few of my favorite foods that taste great and help me stay fit and lose weight:

· Beans, lentils, wild rice, quinoa, soybeans

· Broccoli, artichokes, asparagus, spinach

· Tomatoes, cucumbers, carrots, cabbage

· Almonds, walnuts, pistachios, sunflower seeds

· Apples, bananas, oranges, kiwifruit, papaya

· Water, fruit juice, green tea

· Oatmeal, flax seed

Eating right is a daily activity—so is living a healthy, happy, long and fulfilling life. Sometimes snacks get in the way. The good news is you can always choose to change for the better. I have hundreds of videos that can help at my website, livelife365.com. Hey, they helped me. They can help you too.

peace,

Mike

PERSONAL DEVELOPMENT
I.   MOTIVATION

CHANGE IS GOOD

The other day I dropped my favorite teacup, rendering it no longer a safe or viable receptacle for my daily consumption of my <u>favorite beverage</u>. To say that I was a tad upset is an understatement. I have had that green cup for years, thought of it as kind of a good luck charm, a talisman, if you will; it is even prominently displayed on my website, livelife365. For one awful moment I thought: What am I going to do without my special mug? And then I shook my head and realized how ridiculous I sounded. Eventually I got over my dismay and as I often do, sat down and gave my little ordeal some additional thought. My conclusion was that change, even when it is thrust upon us or may seem bad or ill-timed, is often a good thing.

"Things don't change, we change."~ **Henry David Thoreau**

But for many people, the prospect of change, especially major change, can seem daunting, downright scary, at times. This is a perfectly natural reaction. Why? Because most of us do not like being taken out of our comfort zones. We prefer the mundane routine to the *new* **super** *new* **CHANGE** because our routine is a familiar friend, something that while far from perfect is at least not full of surprises and new challenges. This is okay, unless your desire to do more with yourself and your life.

"If you are not changing, you are not living." ~ **Mike Foster**

Unless we are testing ourselves, trying new things, removing that comfortable routine from our lives, we will never see our greater potential. The best bosses or managers or supervisors or leaders will often place their charges in challenging predicaments just to see how they react, to deem if they have what it takes to be all that they can be. Again, this is not a pleasant or even enjoyable exercise, but it is one that is necessary for self-growth, personal development, and living one's life to its fullest.

"We know what we are, but know not what we may be." ~ **William Shakespeare**

The biggest tragedy is not to have failed or shunned change, but to never

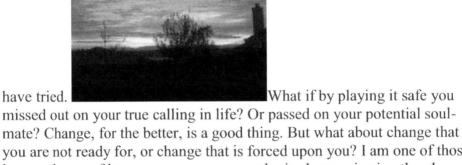

have tried. What if by playing it safe you missed out on your true calling in life? Or passed on your potential soul-mate? Change, for the better, is a good thing. But what about change that you are not ready for, or change that is forced upon you? I am one of those lemonade out of lemons guys, someone who is always viewing the glass as half-full. If change comes and you look at it in a negative light I guarantee that the results will be bad. The good news is that while we may not be able to control the changes headed our way, we can control how we deal with them.

You can't turn on the TV these days without seeing and hearing about how messed up the world is: hunger, war, terrorism, obesity, poverty, global warming, genocide, and just plain uncontrollable anger. How can we change the world when the world's problems seem so vast? The answer is to embrace change and change your self, to look in the mirror and honestly assess your own individual problems and issues and areas in need of improvement. While we may not be able to overcome the seemingly insurmountable problems facing the world, by taking important steps in improving self, the world's issues will be reduced by one.

"Everyone thinks of changing the world, but no one thinks of changing himself." ~ **Tolstoy**

One of the biggest fears facing many people is the fear of failure.

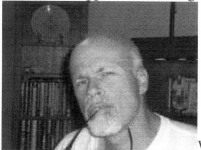 When facing big life changes or just mini-changes that upset the balance of your world, fear of falling flat on your face, of making mistakes, of failure, is natural. The good news: Failure is okay! Why? Because when we fail we are at least trying, and from that effort comes results, feedback from which we can learn, improve, excel.

FAILING = FEEDBACK!

"Anyone who has never made a mistake has never tried anything new." ~ **Albert Einstein**

The other day I thought that my luck had changed in a negative way when I dropped my favorite teacup and was faced with an unexpected change. Instead, I discovered that change, unexpected or planned, big or small, can be a good thing. It all depends on how you embrace it.

peace,

Mike

REWARD YOUR WEAKNESSES (BY TURNING THEM INTO STRENGEHTS)

We all have weaknesses, encompassing myriad aspects of our lives, be it health and fitness challenges, personal development and growth issues, or career and relationship struggles. And then there are food weaknesses. For me, I have a soft spot for salty snacks, like potato chips. I have also been known to power down copious amounts of Doritos with the best of them. What's your food weakness? Candy? Chocolate? Pizza? Cheese? Cake? Soda? Fast food?

The good news is, help is on the way:

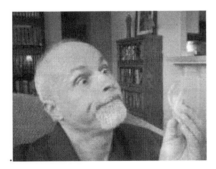

We are, after all, human beings, which makes us flawed individuals, which throughout a lifetime of living leads us to acquire a multitude of weaknesses. Anything from not exercising enough to watching too much daytime TV; from procrastination to condescension. Being too unorganized to being just plain lazy. These are all typical human weaknesses, and all share one commonality:

THEY CAN BE OVERCOME!

"The mind is a terrible thing to waste."

"Mind over matter."

"If you don't mind, it doesn't matter." (one of mine)

"To err is human, to forgive divine."

"Cut yourself some slack, man!" (another one of mine)

By admitting and accepting that as human beings we are going to have our share of weaknesses, we can then begin to understand them, and then work on overcoming them.

Let's return to that potato chip (and Doritos) jones I've been nursing since I tasted my first salty treat as a curious child growing up in New England.

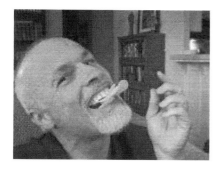

FACT: Chips, while made for the most part from natural ingredients, are loaded with sodium and empty calories.

FACT: Mass consumption of chips will contribute to unhealthy weight gain, hypertension, and a laundry list of assorted maladies (possibly diabetes, heart disease, obesity).

FACT: I love chips and could eat them every day.

SOLUTION: Don't run from your favorite weaknesses, embrace them! Use that weakness as a reward for sacrifice.

Here's where those earlier quotes come into play. Use them to play mind games with yourself. By embracing your weakness as a good thing, you will eliminate some of the guilt associated with that weakness. By denying yourself your weakness (and, granted, this is by far the most difficult part) through self-sacrifice, focusing instead on exercise, moderation, concentration, and good, old-fashion determination during the five-day workweek, you can then reward yourself with that weakness, in moderation, on the weekend.

Make sense?

It's all about risk versus reward. We know what the reward is: taste, comfort, fun, and favorite foods. And I've already listed the risks. The rest is up to you; your choice. While I have focused mainly on food weaknesses, this formula can be used for almost any other weakness; just follow the formula and give it a try.

If you want to live a better, happier, healthier, longer life, then you have to make sacrifices, need to deprive yourself of some things, and then reward yourself for your efforts.

I'd like to close with my favorite quote on this topic, and one I'm the most proud of:

"Exercise control, control your weaknesses, and your weaknesses will become your strengths."

Think about it.

peace,

Mike

SUCCESS IS IN THE EFFORT

Call me old-fashioned, but I enjoy a good sweat, getting my hands dirty and digging into a project; whatever that task or chore may be. And my contentment is not a byproduct of merely completing a job or solving a problem, I also derive great pleasure in the doing, the effort.

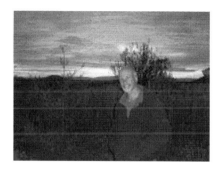

What, you may ask, is old-fashioned about that? Sadly, for many in today's got-to-have-it-now world, plenty.

In a way, we are victims of our technological successes: email, instant messaging, texting, cell phones that connect us to every form of electronic media and communication…especially the Internet. While these amazing innovations have made our lives somewhat easier than they used to be, in return they may have also created more problems than they're worth.

Maybe it's just me, my generation? Or better put: my generation's generation gap.

"Oh, these kids today!" Every generation has adults offering up that lament, for as many diverse reasons as freckles on the sunburned face of a fair-haired teen.

But I see it all the time, from my perspective as a leader at my workplace, to observing my soon-to-be-college-graduated son.

What do I see?

An aversion to that age-old rite of passage in one's life when the youth of the day must pay their dues, start from the bottom and work for peanuts, with the hope and goal, through arduous effort and some luck, of getting somewhere. Hopefully a well-paying job, a satisfying career, but mostly the gratifying feeling of accomplishing something that was worth rolling up those sleeves and breaking a sweat for.

Call is sweat equity or the school of hard knocks. Or how about that good, old-fashioned sensation one derives from enjoying the journey, no matter how long it may be, despite how dire the odds may seem, pursuing a goal that you may or may not attain?

That's what I mean by old-fashioned. Because today's generation looks at me like I suddenly sprouted a third eye in the middle of my face whenever I talk about not just the necessity of effort, but the satisfying feeling said effort brings.

Huh?

What?

Hold on, I'm getting a text…

Okay, what were you saying?

This: No success gained without effort, real effort, is worth having.

And this: No successful individual got that way without first failing: more than likely several times! You can look it up.

If you discover someone who somehow appears to have attained greatness unscathed…look again! Somewhere in that so-called successful person's past, or future, failure lurked and will, no doubt, lurk again.

AND THAT'S A GOOD THING!

Without failure we never learn.

Without failure we do not grow.

Without failure we do not try.

Without failure we do not succeed.

And without effort you will never fail, thus you will never succeed.

All I'm really saying here is:

HARD WORK NEVER HURT ANYONE.

And working hard at something that occupies your mind (and body) in a positive, creative, interesting, challenging, altruistic, humane, productive, and worthwhile way, is the only way you, or anyone, will every become successful. Or fulfilled. Or content.

Or, ultimately, happy.

Work is an integral part of life and without effort you are not alive, not living.

Roll up those sleeves, put your nose to the grindstone, and don't be afraid to get your hands dirty. It will be worth the effort, in more ways that you can imagine.

peace,

Mike

BUILDING SELF-CONFIDENCE

What is confidence? I checked out the definition and one of the reoccurring words used to describe confidence was "belief." Think about that. What is belief but a conviction of one's ideals? You can even toss some faith into the mix.

How does one go about improving their self-confidence? I'm, for the most part, a very self-confident person. Hey, if I wasn't then I bet there would be a good chance that no one would bother to watch any of my self-help videos, or read this blog. But would you believe that, at times, I question my own self-confidence? You bet I do!

The key to success is not in the questioning of one's belief or confidence, but in the understanding that it is okay to do so. And then know what it takes to build that confidence back.

- **SEE YOUR SUCCESS**

One of the things I've practiced over the years is what I call Life Writing. Basically this a version of goal setting, or writing down what I'd like to achieve over the course of a few weeks, months, and even years. A few years ago I was in a rut with my career—I worked at home, telecommuting (which was a good gig for a while), but only using a fraction of my experience. I decided that I wanted to head back into the office, pursue a path that would eventually lead me back into managing people, rather than sitting at a desk at home banging on a keyboard by myself. I literally wrote down what I needed to do to attain this goal, how I was to go about it, what short, mid, and long-terms goals I needed reach in order to succeed. Now, less than 18 months later, I have moved up two levels into management, successfully realizing what I only dreamed (and wrote) about. You can too!

- **RELIVE YOUR SUCCESS**

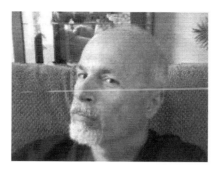

We all have had some modicum of success in our lives, right? Come on, close your eyes and let your imagination roam—see it now? Of course you do. Problem with most folks is they tend to remember to failures more than their successes. Hey, we're human! Whenever I feel my confidence waning, I force my mind to remember a time when I was very successful, encouraging those images and sensations to the forefront of my being, and soon I am basking in my own personal love fest. This is the time to toss the ego out the door. There is nothing wrong with recalling past success to remind yourself that you not only can do the task before you, but **HAVE** done it, or something similar, many times over.

- **PRACTICE YOUR SUCCESS**

Practice may not make perfect, but it sure goes a long way toward making you successful. Sweat equity overcomes myriad other weaknesses. The opposite of success is failure, but failing is not a bad thing. Through failure you learn, get important feedback, and improve. But you have to try and fail first, to be successful, leading to that all important self-confidence. The best athletes are not always those blessed with the best physical gifts. Often, they are the ones who work harder, practice longer, and want it more than the other person. Hard work never hurt anyone; in fact, it just may be the key to improving your confidence.

- **BELIEVE IN YOUR SUCCESS**

There's a fine line between being overconfident and arrogant—believe me, I've walked that tightrope all my life. But I'd rather have too much confidence than too little. My father taught me at a very young age the power of motivation, of positive thinking, of believing that I could do just about anything I put my mind to. And, being young and one who looked up to my old man, I believed him. I've taken that belief in myself with me throughout my life, a life, by the way, filled with as much failure as success. Don't wait for someone else to believe in you, believe in yourself and success may be right around the corner.

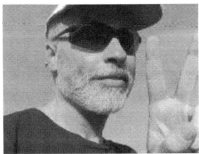

Building self-confidence will not happen overnight—hey, most overnight successes struggled years and years before reaching the top. But it is can be easier than you ever imagined. All you have to do is See, Relive, Practice, and Believe.

Until next time…

peace,

Mike

YOU GOTTA WANT IT

What do the world's most famous athletes, successful businessmen, high-powered politicians, space-traveling astronauts, working actors, creative artists, respected school teachers, and hard-working plumbers all have in 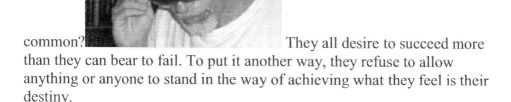 common? They all desire to succeed more than they can bear to fail. To put it another way, they refuse to allow anything or anyone to stand in the way of achieving what they feel is their destiny.

What does this have to do with you? Why, everything, of course. Everything, that is, if you desire to change something about yourself, or have the urge to be something that you currently are not. No matter what your dreams or goals may be—to play left field for the Boston Red Sox or teach high school English—one commonality you must share with anyone who has ever achieved anything worthwhile in this life is the thirst to succeed. The need to overcome any obstacle in your way. But most of all:

YOU GOTTA WANT IT

Just wanting something doesn't mean your work is done, but it does mean that you have taken a giant step toward achieving your goal. This applies to anything you want, from needing the motivation to lose that extra weight you've been trying to lose for years, to finally getting around to figuring out why you detest your job, or your relationships, or your life. Not matter what it is you want to change about yourself or what mountain of opportunity you quest after, you have to want to do it significantly more than not wanting to do it.

I often ask myself what I can do better to help people attain their life goals. I have produced over 350 self-help videos at my website, livelife365.com, and while I have received thousands of encouraging comments and inspirational feedback from successful visitors sharing with me how my websites have helped change their lives for the better, I still want to help thousands (dare I say, millions?) more. One of the biggest roadblocks most people face along the path to success in any worthwhile endeavor is not

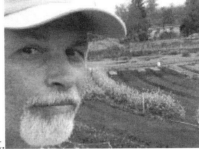

how to start, but *WANTING* to start.

Most people know they have flaws, weaknesses, areas of concern that need to be improved. Though there seems to be an endless supply of informative venues to help most of us—from websites, books, videos, and television shows—none of them will ever work unless someone is ready to change.

I began livelife365.com with one goal in mind: To help as many people as I possibly could change their lives for the better. One of the first videos I produced was one of me sitting in my office, surrounded by books, talking about the significance of not only recognizing the need to change, but the vital importance of *WANTING* to change. I recently received a nice comment on that video, prompting me to watch it again, and, guess what? While a little longer than I would like it to be, the message was still strong…and important. So much so I was motivated to write this article with you in the hopes that it may be that one little push to give you the direction or desire you have been missing and looking for.

Personal development, self-growth, achieving goals, pursuing your dreams, and changing your life for the better are never easy. It takes hard work, direction, patience, but most of all it takes desire and determination so strong that you refuse to allow anything or anyone to stand in the way of what it is you want to do.

YOU GOTTA WANT IT!

May you achieve all that you desire and deserve.

peace,

Mike

TURN BAD HABITS INTO GOOD ONES

I recently received an email from someone who had visited my video site, livelife365.com. After viewing my video on how to beat addictions, she wanted to share with me her own recent success in overcoming her struggles with alcohol, and then ask me if I had any advice for helping her overcome her ongoing addiction to cigarettes. I offered several successful methods and programs that helped me quit smoking (years and years ago, thank goodness), and then added one of my favorite sayings:

TURN BAD HABITS INTO GOOD ONES!

While far from a cure-all, especially while attempting to quit smoking cigarettes (nicotine addiction is one of the most difficult battles to overcome), this advice has helped me change my life for the better time and time again.

Using smoking as an example, what I suggested to my email friend was to stop cold turkey. Actually, I suggested that she check with her medical professional first before making any drastic lifestyle change in diet, fitness or addictions. Once she stopped smoking she should then replace that nasty habit with a healthier one—like exercise. Start off slowly at first (a walking program is always my first choice for those just beginning to get back into an exercise routine), and then build from there. I then suggested eating healthier foods. Essentially, what this does is force you to stay away from the butts. By introducing healthy habits into your life, your mind and body (and don't forget the other member of the triad of balance, the spirit) will rebel against such a negative intrusion—like inhaling burning tobacco leaves into your once pink lungs, introducing a toxic poison that will cut years off your precious life. After a while, not only will your body reject tobacco (or alcohol or greasy fast-foods), but your mind and spirit will too.

I am a huge believer that diet and exercise, along with a positive mental approach, can cure just about anything. Most of the good habits I recommended to combat the struggle with quitting nicotine addiction can be applied to other bad habits as well—be it trying to stop the over-consumption of alcohol or attempting to cut down on fast-foods or soda.

I used to be a Diet Coke fiend. Let me give you some background about myself first. I was once a heavy drinker, from the age of sixteen to thirty-six. I figure I used up all of my booze tickets in twenty years, when they should have lasted me a lifetime. Using the bad habits/good habits method, along with other effective programs, I was able to quit drinking, and haven't touched the hard stuff in over fifteen years. But one habit I acquired, after giving up the vodka, was soda. Diet Coke, to be precise.

Figuring I had eliminated just about all other vices from my life, what harm could soda do me, right? Especially diet soda. I used to suck down five, six, seven or more bottles a day for years…until I started reading up on what was actually in diet soda. Along with the high sodium, which causes bloating, and various gastrointestinal side effects, overconsumption of diet soda is far from a healthy beverage option.

The solution: Turn that bad habit into a good one. My good one was: green tea. Never that much of a coffee drinker, I had read about the health benefits of drinking green tea, so I tried it—and have enjoyed it ever since.

This method can be applied to just about any bad habit. Watching too much bad TV? Shut off the set (there are some good shows on television, but it's up to you to find them and then only watch the good ones) and pick up a good habit—like reading. Or a fun or interesting hobby. Relationship with your spouse getting dull? Spice it up or switch things around. Some of our routines, while necessary and comforting, can become ruts, if we allow them to. Turn that bad habit into a good one.

As I have said, this is not a cure-all for whatever ails you (some problems need bigger solutions), but give this method a try and see for yourself. The results may surprise you.

Good luck with whatever challenges you face. And may all your habits be good ones.

peace,

Mike

A LIFE WITHOUT GOALS IS A LIFE UNFULFILLED

I didn't want to write this post. Not because I don't have a passion for the subject matter—I live for goals! I just didn't feel like sitting here, pen in hand vexing my brain into coming up with today's post. But here I am, writing about the necessity of goals in our lives, despite desiring to be elsewhere. Why? Because I have to—it's one of my goals.

Recently, I decided that I would write three blog posts a week—on Monday, Wednesday, and Friday. I visit dozens of blogs each day, taking note of content, style, and frequency of posts, and based on that figured that three was just about right. That number also fit in with my wanting to write about the three main themes of livelife365—Health, Personal Development, and Entertainment—each week. After making this decision, I then made it a goal. Being serious about my goals, and today being Friday, I felt compelled, bound by self-promise, to keep my word to myself. Ah, goals!

I am a firm believer that to be successful in life one needs to have a plan. Now, I also understand the need for spontaneity and that I am unable to "control" a lot of situations, realize that life often tosses us curveballs of fate, both ominous and serendipitous, that my plans or goals make little dent in. For that I like to say, "Worry about the things you can control and not about what you cannot." What I am getting at is the gist of this post, and that is: Take charge of your life by setting goals!

SHORT-RANGE GOALS

Let's say you're trying to lose weight—I strongly suggest setting a weekly goal for which to strive. For me, when I lost 40 pounds in six months, I set a goal of losing two pounds a week as something to shoot for. My short-range goals also included weighing myself daily, keeping a diet journal of everything I put in my mouth, and counting calories consumed and burned. A lot of effort, but well worth it—it worked!

Set clearly defined goals, but make sure they are not too easy or too difficult to attain. If they are too easy, then raise the bar; find yourself something worthwhile to shoot for. But don't raise that bar too high—if a goal appears unattainable, then you begin to lose faith, get frustrated, regress, and sometimes give up. It is a challenging balancing act, but if you put some thought and effort into it, you'd be surprised at how effective your results will be.

Speaking of effort—setting, maintaining, and reaching goals is all about effort. Hard work. You will get out of it only what you put into it. If you are serious about changing your life for the better—physically, intellectually, financially, spiritually, relationship-wise—and bringing more purpose and fulfillment into your days, it takes some work. Work well worth the effort. But you need a plan. You need goals.

MID-RANGE GOALS

Have you ever sat in a job interview, or maybe just a performance review with your boss, and heard this query: "Where do you see yourself in five years?" Big groan, right?

Most of us are just trying to survive today, or at least this week, month, maybe year. Think about five years for a moment—it seems like a long time, but, for me, at least, these last five years have flown by! If you are not where you want to be now, chances are you did not give enough attention to your goals five years ago—make sense? Put another way: If you see yourself five years from now in a better career, nicer home, married with children (or divorced, free, and consuming fruity beverages on a beach in the Caribbean), you will need to start planning NOW. Start setting goals.

- Make a list of your dreams and goals
- Make a plan of how to attain the above
- Set a doable timetable
- Put forth the effort
- Remember that there will be snags, forks in the road, challenges and adversity along the way, so…
- Don't be afraid to reassess, tweak, and refresh your goals. As you evolve, so do your goals.
- Stay the course, never give up, dream, and live!

LONG-RANGE GOALS

When I think long-range, I think ten years or more, maybe longer. What I'm really trying to say is—when can I retire? And: how much money will I need? Also where?

A few years ago, I made a major commitment and decisions that would greatly determine when and how well my wife and I would retire and live. How did I go about doing this? I set goals. Sensing I was nearing the end of my prime earning years, I made a concerted effort to work more hours, earn more money, so we could save more. I set short- and mid-range goals for contributions in our 401k plans, upping the percentages each year until we eventually hit our maxes. I reworked our budget to help meet these goals (a good practice to do at least once a year), cutting spending here, sacrificing there, without compromising our other goal of enjoying our lives today.

These are just some of my goals. Your goals will be different, and they will need different strategies and planning. No matter what your dream life is, what goals you need to work on to achieve it, the more effort you put forth the better your results will be. Focus, plan, work hard, and you're on your way.

Set goals and stick with them and your dream life, before you know it, will become reality.

Remember: A life without goals is a life unfulfilled.

Wow, for a guy who didn't feel like writing, I sure wrote a lot. Why? Because it was a goal.

peace,

Mike

LIFE BLOCKAGE

Has this ever happened to you? One day, you're doing your thing—whatever that thing may be—you know, taking care of business, tending to the daily details of your life. It's a breeze, a walk in the park, a nice, comfortable routine that you enjoy. Sure, it can be mundane, at times, a bit of the same old/same old, but it's a smooth, effortless ride. You're getting stuff done. You're productive. Happy. Living la dolce vida (and maybe even la vida loca, for you Ricky Martin fans out there). And then, out of nowhere, out of the blue, it all ends. Stops. Ceases to not only be fun, but to be at all. You are suddenly stuck. In a rut.

BLOCKED!

This sensation can apply to just about any situation in anyone's life. As a writer, the first thing that comes to mind is: Writer's Block. I can hear the moans and screams from my fellow writer's out there—no, no, not that! Not writer's block! Do not go there!

Okay, I won't, not just yet. Instead, how about I go here: constipation.

Now we're talking about some serious blockage.

Isn't that a bit of a stretch, Mike? From writer's block to constipation?

Not really. Here's why: to avoid any kid of blockage in your life (let's call this Life Blockage), you need to follow a few simple tips—plan ahead, practice good, healthy routines, balance your triad—mind, body, and spirit, and work hard at it. Every day.

Life blockage isn't limited to writer's block or your ability or inability to regulate your bowels. It can challenge your relationships or careers, appear as a mid-life crisis, and mess with your diet and health; just about anything in your life. The good news: working on these tips can help you manage most of what life, and life blockage, sends your way.

DO IT EVERY DAY

It is said that practice makes perfect. While seeking perfection can be a practice in futility, practicing is a good thing. To get better at anything, you need to work at it. Repetition is an important key on the road to improvement, but mistakes are bound to happen—another good thing. Making mistakes is encouraged, as long as you learn from them.

Let's go back and take a look at writing again. I strongly suggest you write every day. Easy, right, you're a writer. But it is easier said than done—at least for me it is. I mean, who has anything relevant to say every day? Not a lot of people. But you still need to write, all the time, if your desire is to become a good writer, and to improve your writing skills. So write. Every day. At times (lots of times) you will write bad prose and you will discard most of what you have toiled hours to create. If you want to write (and those who really want to write, will write—it's almost an unstoppable compulsion) you will, and, if I may be so bold, you will enjoy the process.

Writing every day will keep the writer's block away!

Using these methods will help you with most any challenges life tosses your way.

- Work at (_____) every day
- Understand that it is okay, encouraged even, to make mistakes
- Learn from those mistakes
- Work smart

Working smart is managing your time, balancing your tasks, and doing the little things that you learn and pick up along the way. One of the tips I picked up to help me combat the evils of writer's block was writing every day. And on those days when your creative muse is your best friend, take a moment to jot down all those amazing ideas that seem to be overflowing from your brain. You will be grateful for them a few weeks later when your brain bogs down and is as productive as a wedge of Swiss cheese.

Another tip that is great for writers and writer's block is to read, all the time, everything you can get your hands on. Diverse data, fiction and non-fiction, books and magazines, every day. **READ**.

The more you know, the more you can write about.

So, what does any of this have to do with, you know, ahh, that other backed up situation I mentioned earlier?

Constipation?

Yup, that's the one.

Apply the same tips.

- Work at it every day. This means eating the right foods and the right amounts, along with an exercise program
- Make mistakes and learn from them. Discover which foods make your plumbing happy and which ones do not. I can give you a one-word hint—FIBER! Lots of fruits and veggies. And stay away from cheese and processed foods.
- Work smart—see above

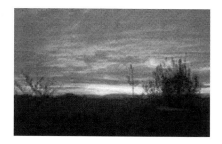

When I sat down to write this, I was blocked—just my mind, not anywhere else. My life these days has been filled with more than my share of outside distractions and challenges that have upset my routines and balance, creating a blockage. A life blockage.

Whenever I am faced with these challenges, these life blockages, I always fall back on the common sense methods that have helped me overcome myriad difficulties in the past. Writing down a few of them in this post reminded, and reassured, me that they still are effective. Still work for me.

I hope they work for you too.

peace,

Mike

JUST DO IT—10 TIPS TO GET YOU STARTED

We've all heard those three words before, right? Just do it. And while I encourage taking personal accountability for your actions, and further support the notion that we **DO**, indeed, control a lot of our life, getting from the **WANTING** to do it to the **DO** of doing it is a different story.

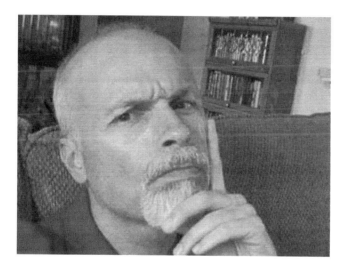

And it isn't about the *HOW* of just doing it. I have an entire <u>videography</u> filled with tips and proven methods and programs that explain, in detail, **HOW** to lose weight, battle addictions, get in shape, balance your life, and much more. I have written extensively about the same topics.

Google <u>"weight loss"</u> and you will get 93 million responses offering ways to lose as much weight in as short a time as you want, need, desire, or dream. The **HOW**, while at times different and debatable, is not always the issue.

Of course, I'd like to think that my methods for weight loss, eating a <u>high-fiber diet</u> and <u>making your calories count,</u> are more effective than what all those other sites are offering (they are), but if you are not **READY** and **WILLING** to just **DO** it, no diet or exercise program will work. **NONE**.

But I have good news for you: helpful tips to motivate you from *WANTING* to do it to just *DOING* it.

TEN TIPS TO GET YOU STARTED.

1. ENVISION THE NEW YOU

Let's say you're trying to lose weight. Try taping an inspiring photo on your fridge or workstation of you in that nice bathing suit you would love to fit in again. See your future! This works for anything: new car, flat screen TV, house! If you stare at your dreams every day, something may just "click" in your brain, and help motivate you to take that first step.

2. REPROGRAM YOUR BRAIN

You have the power to do more than you think. Start thinking differently about the way your mind looks at:

- Food (if you're trying to lose weight or eat better)
- Exercise (if you're working on getting back in shape)
- Finances (balancing your budget, trying to get out of debt)

Change your mind and you can change your life.

3. REALIZE THAT IT'S OKAY TO FAIL

Oft times failure is good. Why? Because it means you're at least trying, attempting something. Failing = Feedback. The only people who never fail are the ones who never try to do anything.

4. EDUCATE YOURSELF

You already have a good start toward this, but read *more*. Read, research, watch, listen. Knowledge is power. If you want to lose weight or eat healthier or quit smoking or balance your life livelife365 is a great place to start, but don't stop here.

5. DISCOVER SUPPORT GROUPS

During your self-education, besides discovering sites like livelife365.com, you will also find lots of other wonderful support groups of like-minded thinkers. Don't limit your support groups to just online ones: investigate local and community groups and clubs. Remember, they call them "support" groups for a reason.

6. TAKE BABY STEPS

A little at a time goes a long way. If you're trying to quit smoking, cutting down from three packs a day to only ten cigarettes is progress. Don't take on more than you can handle; this leads to discouragement, which can lead to giving up. Like that toddler learning to walk, you may fall on your bottom a few times, but, just like a kid, you need to get right back up and keep going...taking one baby step at a time.

7. DON'T LET ANYONE STAND IN YOUR WAY

Hey, it's your life, right? If it is your desire to drop a few (or a lot) of pounds or stop drinking or smoking, then why allow anyone (or anything) to get in the way of your goals. It is imperative that your significant other, family, and friends are all on board; if not, at least don't allow them to deter you from your desires. If they care about you, they will understand.

8. IF NOT FOR YOU, THEN FOR THEM

If your six-year-old asks why you smoke after their teacher told the class that smoking is bad for you, what do you say to that child? If *you* don't care about your health, think about how your sudden death or lengthy illness would affect your loved ones.

9. HIT BOTTOM

Sadly, sometimes it takes a life-changing event before we finally take life-changing actions. Believe me, I know. I was divorced twice, addicted to nicotine and alcohol, bankrupt and depressed before I finally hit bottom and decided to do something about it. I strongly suggest not waiting for the bottom--start now!

10. CONSIDER THE ALTERNATIVE

You may never hit bottom, never take action. If this is the case, what's left? Obesity, heart disease, diabetes, and cancer are the leading causes of death in the world today. The sad fact is that most of those deaths can be prevented by taking action *NOW* by changing your lifestyle from harmful to healthy.

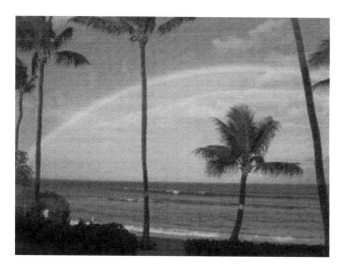

When someone tells you to **JUST DO IT**, they are trying to help you, trying to motivate you into challenging and changing yourself into living a long, happy, healthy, productive life.

Livelife365 is here to help you **DO** just that.

I sincerely hope I have motivated you to try to...

JUST DO IT.

peace,

Mike

THE CYNICAL OPTIMIST

Is your glass half-full?

Or is the grass always greener on the other side of the street? Do you feel that no matter what happens, as long as you try your hardest, do your best, be kind to others and think nice thoughts, things will work out? Or do you feel that it doesn't matter what you do, bad things, eventually, will happen to good people. Maybe you think that all politicians are crooks; bankers and lawyers too? And the government—they don't really care about us, they are just hanging around taking kickbacks and creating and covering up scandals, right? Perhaps that's being too…what? Cynical? Or am I being too optimistic? Jeez, I can't win!

Maybe that's it—we just can't win!

That's crazy, of course you can, you just have to keep on keeping on and put your nose to the grindstone. It will all work out in the end—time heals all wounds, right?

The heck with time: what about all the world's problems—hunger, war, terrorism, racism, unaffordable health care, unemployment, corruption, apathy!

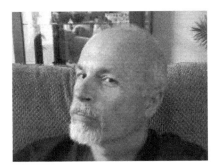

Okay, but what about the miracle of watching your child come into the world, the awesome naked beauty of a sunset, the natural sensation you get from laughing so hard that tears streak your cheeks?

Tears are right! I feel like crying whenever I think about not having a job, the cost of gasoline, the jokers in Washington (and Europe), and my child support payments!

Tears of joy for having the ability to earn a living, being able to afford to own a car that you can drive across this amazing country; the freedom to choose your leaders, vote for change, and the blessing given to you to have the opportunity to raise a child.

Man, talk about a cockeyed optimist!

Boy, what a negative cynic!

Who am I describing? Anyone you know? Or do the above diatribes hit closer to home?

Are you one of those people who believes that every day brings with it the opportunity to do something incredible?

Or one that dreads waking up to another miserable twenty-fours of getting stepped on, tossed aside, paranoid that someone is going to do something bad to you?

Me? I like to think that good things will happen to me—and you too!—if I put a positive spin on everything in my life. In fact, I strongly believe that a good mental attitude, filled with positive energy and happy thoughts, goes a long way toward a healthy, happy, fulfilling life.

Yeah, but what about—

I know, I know, there is a lot of bad in the world, lots of heartache and pain; suffering. And there are often terrible and unavoidable pitfalls and horrors that befall each and every one of us, sometimes daily or weekly—certainly several times throughout our lives.

Guess what? It's called **LIFE**. And **LIFE** happens, with us out without us.

"Life is the definition of imperfection."

- Mike Foster

You can't have a gorgeous sunset without clouds, can't put a roof over your head without cutting down some trees, and cannot live life without a few (or several) tough breaks occurring along the way.

The key to a successful, happy, healthy life is staring at you in the mirror every morning when you brush those choppers—you. I'm not saying turn your back on your problems, or ignore the atrocities that afflict millions of innocent human beings by just smiling at the new day and hoping for the best.

What I'm saying is we all have a choice, to either find that happiness, that hope that resides in us all. Or embrace the darkness, the negativity, that cynicism that lives within us too.

And even if you are faced with seemingly insurmountable odds, have to deal with daily drudgery and setbacks; even if your life, or a loved one's life, seems destined to turn into nothing but bad luck and heartache, you, too, have a choice.

Deal, cope, survive.

Smile, love, live.

Am I as hopeful and cheerful and optimistic as I can be all the time? No. Do I sometimes fall victim of feeling victimized, or think that the world, and my little slice of it, seems hopeless and a waste of time? Sometimes, but, thankfully, not very often.

The key, again, is right inside your head, your heart, your soul. And embracing the wonderful paradox derived from living each moment, striving for the best possible existence, every day in every way.

peace,

Mike

ACCENTUATE THE POSITIVE

I recently wrote an article called the cynical optimist, where I noted the sometimes paradoxical challenges we all face when confronted by daily life circumstances. That choice being to accept said task or chore or adversity in an open, positive, optimistic way. Or look down at it like it is something that your foot just stepped in, another one of life's ongoing jokes and misadventures that seem aimed directly at you.

I still believe that we can choose to be happy, and in effect, positive, if we will our minds to do so. Now, I'm not saying that if you get run over by a bus and are lying in a pool of blood on the interstate and some negative thoughts may seep (along with that blood) into your mind that you should ignore your injuries and smile, whistle, and watch the birdies tweeting around your concussive skull. But I am saying that, yes, even while you are being strapped to a gurney and being shoved into the back end of an ambulance, yes, even then, you still have the option to choose optimism over cynicism.

Wow, some happy joker this guy is, huh?

Yes, for the most part. Why? Because it's just as easy to choose to be positive as it is to embrace negativity...and it's far healthier.

One of the keys to success and happiness is not only cultivating a positive attitude and persona, but reinforcing that attitude every day. Most of us enjoy positive feedback, whenever we receive it. But those platitudes and kudos are not always available. What to do...?

Give yourself positive reinforcement. Give yourself a pat on the back for the job well done if your manager or supervisor or boss does not. Only, of course, if you deserve one.

If you do something wrong, make a mistake, fail, it's not the end of the world. Rather, it is an opportunity to learn, grow, achieve. Then reinforce whatever positive success factors gained from the experience.

Remember, we can choose, for the most part, to be positive throughout our daily existence, no matter how difficult that can be at times. But more importantly, we also need to reinforce this positivity with encouraging reminders, daily affirmations, and well-earned acclamation.

If we are constantly reminded that we have had past successes during certain endeavors, then we take from those positive memories the encouragement and experience necessary for continued success.

Think about it.

peace,

Mike

PERSONAL DEVELOPMENT
II.   INSPIRATION

\

IS LIVE WORTH LIVING?

The other day, I received an email from a recent visitor to livelife365. I get my share of comments and feedback and welcome them in any form, especially from those seeking my advice or requesting a special video just for them. This particular email was from a young man in his late teens, a difficult time in a young man's life, for sure, often fraught with confusion and questions. In his email, he questioned the purpose of living a healthy life, while denying oneself many of the excessive vices that we all are tempted by, when, in the end, we all are going to die anyway. In essence, he asked:

Is Life Worth Living?

My teenaged friend offers up a good point: Why, indeed, should we exercise, maintain a healthy weight, and eschew excess, when we are all stamped with a termination date? The answer seems obvious, but it is not. I should know, for I have, in the past, abused alcohol, drugs, food, tobacco, and life. I have lived that unfulfilled life, that life with little or no purpose other than to sate one's desires, to grab as much gusto as possible without care for the repercussions. And you know what? I didn't like it, wasn't productive, and, most certainly, was not enjoying my life, nor living up to my potential.

Why? Because we are put here for a reason. I firmly believe that each one of us has a specific purpose that we must pursue throughout our lifetimes, be it a few years or ten decades. I also feel that to not do this is in essence wasting one's life. It is not only vital to live your life to its fullest every day, seeking your true reason for being, but it is your obligation as a human being. It is what separates us from all other species that inhabit this planet.

Bringing me back to the letter that inspired this post:

<u>Is Life Worth Living?</u>

I say, yes, of course, it has to be, right? But for too many it just may not be. One of the motivating reasons behind *livelife365.com* , was the prospect of being able to reach as many people as possible, many of them questioning their purpose in life or needing assistance with weight loss or nutritional advice, and then being able to help them change their lives. Helping them see that their time on earth is valuable and precious. Helping them live life every day in every way.

I like to say that **Your Life is a Novel; Make it a Good One**. We all know the difference between reading a good book and a bad one. Our life, like a good novel, should be filled with so much purpose on every page that you can't wait to see what happens next, while savoring what just transpired.

The French have an expression: *Raison d'etre*. It simply means: Reason For Being.

Once you find your reason for being, whatever it is, you will find your answer to the question: **Is Life Worth Living?**

I look at the young man who wrote to me questioning his own reason for being as an inspiration, a reminder of what my *raison d'etre* is. I feel that I have been put on this earth to assist as many people as possible, helping them achieve their life goals along the road to personal development and self-improvement. Whether with a laugh or a pat on the back, a self-deprecating anecdote or inspired moment from my past that I can share, I feel that it is my duty as a human being, my purpose, to help others improve their lives.

We only have one life, one chance to do something with our short time on earth, one opportunity that should never, ever be taken for granted or wasted. Am I saying life is all hard work and no fun? No, not at all, but life takes a lot of effort and sacrifice to be successful and fulfilled. The key is moderation and finding the balance, along with continuous self-study and research; oh, and don't forget to have some fun along the way. No one said it was easy, but I will say that if you work hard each day the benefits will far outweigh the effort.

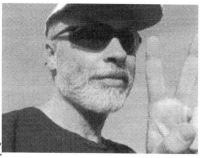

Is Life Worth Living?

I hope I have answered that question in the most positive fashion. Keep living your life, every day in every way.

peace,

Mike

FIND YOUR SPIRITUALITY

When we talk about spirituality, most people automatically think of faith, their high power, and their feelings about their god of choice.

While I find all of that very spiritual, I feel that spiritually is so much more; it has to be. Why? Because to be in total harmonious balance, to be a complete human being, we have to be physically fit and healthy, mentally strong and focused, *and* spiritually sound. To limit one's spiritual health to just having faith, higher powers, and communal worship is akin to running ten miles a day then smoking a pack of cigarettes—something's missing.

I am constantly searching for that inner peace, that tranquil happiness, that meditative state that I feel only total spirituality can give us. Again, going to a place of worship every week, celebrating with like people, and practicing one's faith is a good thing…I just feel we have to do more to be more.

For me, finding one's spirituality is a daily activity, just as working on my mind and body, and improving my triad of balance is.

Ten Ways To Find Your Spirituality

1. Take A Walk In The Wilderness. For me, there's nothing better than getting out and communing with nature, away from the noises and distractions of the busy world (and your busy life). Find a tranquil spot that you can share with the birds and squirrels and you will find yourself.

2. Exercise The Mind And Body. To achieve balance in my life, I need for my mind and body and spirit to be aligned. What better way to strengthen one than by working on the others. Working up a sweat, for me, is a natural spiritual high; as is working a crossword puzzle. Work the mind and body, and the spirit will come around.

3. Reach Out And Touch Someone. When was the last time you received a hug? Or initiated one? Hopefully it was as recently as today. Physical contact with another human being (or even a dog or cat, to a lesser extent) is not only spiritually uplifting, but an essential necessity for happiness and spiritual wholeness.

4. Be Kind. One of my favorite adages is: Do onto others as you would want them to do onto you. Good vibes are contagious. What goes around comes around. Spread joy and you shall be joyous. A smile goes a lot farther than a snarl. Random acts of kindness should be second nature for us

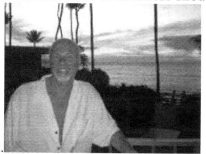

all. Think about it.

5. Live In The Moment. I am a planner, a multitasker, a busy guy with lots of irons in the fire. I often have to force myself to slow down, take a breath, stop and enjoy what is happening in the here and now, and not what needs to be done in the then and when. Enjoy the ride, the process, the journey…the moment.

6. Keep Busy. An idle mind is the devil's playground. While it is good to live in the moment, it is also very good to have lots to do. That doesn't mean to never chill out, take a vacation or relax. It just means to have some hobbies, a few vocations, careers, goals, things to do. Every day, as much as your schedule permits. The more the merrier, as long as they are positive endeavors that add to your personal resume as a complete, happy, fulfilled person.

7. Give Of Yourself. When I help someone less fortunate than myself it makes me feel good—and it should! There's nothing wrong with feeling good when you've done a good deed. Just don't make that the main motivation for doing it. Do it because to not do it would be as unnatural as not eating, or breathing.

8. Hang Up The Phone! Living with all of the amazing innovations in this technological age is something I never would have dreamed of twenty years ago. But too much of a good thing can turn into a bad thing. I spend way too many hours in front of my computer out of the necessity of having to earn a living and passion for my website, but I shut it off as often as I can. You should too. Toss the cell, pull the plug on that iPod, stop texting, switch the TV off, and find a quiet spot to reflect, think, meditate…live. You will be happy you did.

9. Keep The Faith. Believe in yourself as much as your higher power. Go to your place of worship and sing the praises of your faith. Share your feelings with those like-minded people and your spirits will soar. No matter what floats your boat or makes you happy, faith is a good thing; it is the foundation of spirituality.

10. Stay Positive. These days the news, at times, can bring you down, test your spirit, your happiness. But the good thing is: we can choose to be happy, to be positive. Why would anyone choose otherwise? Even when times seem darkest, when life is at its worst, opting to be positive, to see the glass as half full, is still a personal choice. Choose to be positive and good things will not only follow, but it will be one giant step toward finding your spirituality.

These were just a few of the many activities and practices I follow as I constantly work at improving my spirituality. I hope some of them work for you. I would love for you to share some of yours with me.

peace,

Mike

WITHOUT HOPE, WE HAVE NOTHING

While researching this post, I encountered so many excellent, usable quotes that I had to stop for a second and further ponder why I desired to write a post about a topic that has already been written about extensively.

I mean, the current president of these United States of America, Barrack Obama, practically based his entire candidacy on hope, or better put: on the premise, and promise, of believing in and rediscovering a lost hope. He even penned a best-selling book called "The Audacity of Hope." One of his heroes, Martin Luther King, Jr., constantly orated about hope:

"If you lose hope, somehow you lose the vitality that keeps life moving, you lose that courage to be, that quality that helps you go on in spite of it all. And so today I still have a dream."

Men and women throughout history talk of hope, the opposite of despair, which is also a highly quoted subject matter. Hope and despair are forever linked; you can't think about one without thinking about the other. The great writer, George Bernard Shaw, may have put it best:

"He who has never hoped can never despair."

And for those who like their hope quotes a bit darker, there's always that cheery, optimistic philosopher Freidrich Nietzsche:

"Hope is the worst of evils, for it prolongs the torments of man."

Although I prefer a softer, kinder hope, as I mentioned earlier, *"Ya can't talk hope without talking about the bad stuff too."* (One of my quotes. Don't think it will be enshrined into the quote Hall of Fame anytime soon).

One of the things that continually amazes me is the hope I witness in others who have no business believing in anything, much less hope. It makes little difference what specific hardship or malady, act of violence or bad luck I am referring to, only that these brave, resilient souls somehow find it within themselves to persevere, to go on and rise above whatever tragedy that has befallen them and do something with their lives. Which, as always, brings me to what I'm all about—what livelife365.com is all about: living life every day in every way and not letting anyone or anything stand in your way.

Which also brings me to this amazing email I received from a loyal follower of livelife365. His name is Pierre and he is a lot like you, me, and millions of other people in this world. He is a human being and he's made mistakes, embraced vices like smoking (cigarettes and marijuana), overeating, and practicing bad nutritional habits, which means he is not perfect, just like you and me. But like those aforementioned folks who refuse to give up even while facing great odds, Pierre wanted to change his life for the better. He began by researching green tea, because he had heard that drinking green tea was a good way to lose weight. He found my green tea video on YouTube, and then, like many others, stumbled upon my site, and began watching my videos on weight loss, diet and nutrition, and motivation. And, according the Pierre, livelife365 helped him lose 18 pounds in three months and changed his life.

Like I've said countless times, there are hundreds of thousands of Pierre's out there that need to change their lives for the better. All they need is a push in the right direction and some common sense advice on how to do it. I strongly feel livelife365 can offer that push and advice.

In closing, I leave you with a quote from one of the most quoted political figures of the last century, Winston Churchill:

"The pessimist sees difficulty in every opportunity. The optimist sees the opportunity in every difficulty."

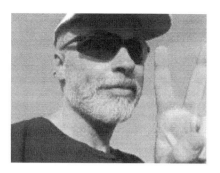

peace (and hope),

Mike

FINDING SELF BY LOSING SELF

I recently started meditating, counting my breath, sitting in a quiet room and trying not to think about anything. And you know something? It's not as easy as it sounds. In fact, you try it. Try sitting still, with your legs folded over each other, your eyes half-closed and unfocused, willing your mind to banish any outside thoughts from entering it. Go ahead, I'll wait.

You probably discovered very quickly that thoughts, distractions and outside interferences overwhelm your ability to focus, to render your mind a blank slate, to meditate on nothing. And that's okay, I warned you that it was challenging, maybe even impossible, at first. But that's not the point of why I meditate, why I sit in a room by myself and try to focus on nothing. I do so to find self. And I have discovered, through trial and error, research and reading, that to find self you have to first lose self.

Huh?

"Huh?" is right. But it's a good kind of huh, one that makes you think, makes you take note, makes you intrigued, I hope. Makes you want to read on.

I often talk about the **TRIAD OF BALANCE**, what I refer to as the continuous process of maintaining the harmonic balance between the mind, body, and spirit. I have found that when I have all three of these essentials working and in harmony with one another, then I am at my strongest and happiest, enjoying the most effective way of living my life to its fullest. If one of my big three is out of whack, but the other two are still strong, while I may feel a bit off and not my complete self, I can still do most of what I need to do…only not all of what I want to do to be all that I need to be. That is why finding that balance, working on the mind, body, and spirit all the time, is one of the main focuses in my life, this blog, and a driving force for livelife365.

So to strengthen my spiritual side, after working, of course, on my intellectual and physical areas, I decided I needed to lose self first…to find self later.

Okay, Mike, how does one lose self?

Glad you asked. Meditation is a good start. Let's go back to trying not to allow any thoughts to invade your mind while you sit still with your eyes

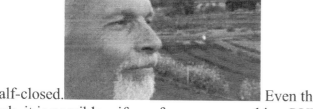

half-closed. Even though this is a difficult task, it is possible…if you focus on everything *BUT* your own thoughts while doing it.

Ummm, you lost me.

Got back to your quiet place, sit, focus, and try not to think. Only this time, if a thought tries to weasel its way into your mind, just gently push it aside. Then, while trying not to let *YOUR* thoughts back in, allow your mind the freedom to let everything else in.

Huh?

Hold on, I'm getting there. Notice your surroundings. The sound of the clock on the wall, the wind rustling the leaves or tinkling your wind chimes. A car passing by. Your refrigerator rumbling into life. Everything else but *YOUR* thoughts. Make sense?

Kind of. But what's the point?

The point is, by allowing the outside world in, while trying to eliminate your internal thoughts, you have, in a small way, lost your self. And this, in a larger sense, helps you find your self.

Finding self goes a long way toward <u>finding your spirituality</u>.

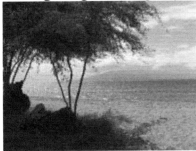And that helps balance your triad.

peace,

Mike

YOUR TIME ON EARTH

How much time do any of us have? Time on earth? Eight decades, if we're lucky, maybe nine? When you're in your twenties, eighty or ninety years of life seems like a lot of time, doesn't it? And it is, I guess, from a twenty-something's point of view. How about for folks like myself, in their early 50's? Eighty years looks a bit less large. In fact, it looks like a number that is fast approaching and too close to just around the corner.

No matter your age or how eighty or ninety years looks to you in the scheme of things, the purpose of this blog entry (and the attached video, for those who prefer watching and listening versus reading) is to emphasize the importance of time. More to the point: our time on earth. Because no matter if you live to 100 or leave this rock way too early, the thing that will shape your days while alive, as well as fill those days with purpose and meaning, is what you do along the way. What you do each and every day.

Life is precious. Like is boring. Life is amazing. Life is difficult. Life is fun. Life is horrible. Life is happy. Life is sad. Life is the most beautiful thing in the world. Life...is life. There are things that occur every second in this world that make us cringe, shake our heads, cry, and wonder how this could possibly be happening. And yet during that same day, if we are lucky, life will show us how utterly wonderful it is: a cute puppy, a random act of kindness or heroism, a stunning sunset, the love of another human being. My point is this: no matter what life is handing you or how the problems of the world make you feel, you have an obligation to yourself, to the rest of the six billion souls who inhabit this planet. You have to try. Work hard. Strive to be the best you can be. Be kind, caring, considerate. Work to right wrongs, help others, set a good example. But mostly, you have to make YOUR LIFE as complete and fulfilling as possible. By doing all that YOU can to make a difference, to leave a positive mark, to grow and learn and take personal accountability for your actions, to balance your mind, body, and spirit, you are taking care of self. And if everyone did just that--made themselves the best person possible--the world would be that much better a place. Now I'm not saying all that is wrong with this world will suddenly be right, but a lot of it will be. Think about it.

But remember, be it ten years or one hundred, this is YOUR time on earth. And what I feel when I think about that is this: I do not want to waste it. I will not allow anyone or anything to stand in the way of all I want to do during my time here. I embrace this time on earth because it is MY time; as it is YOUR time. And as for me, I want to leave a mark, a legacy, a positive impact. Make my eight or nine, hopefully, ten decades the best they can be. And when I close my eyes at night and it's just me and my higher power, I want to be able to say that I worked hard every day, tried to make a difference, helped others as best I could, and lived my life during my time here on earth to its fullest. And I want you to be able to do the same.

Peace,

Mike

LIFE'S TOO SHORT...

Whenever I pick up a new book to read I am very happy, drunk with anticipation that this new venture into this writer's mind will be a trip well worth the effort and investment. As a book collector and bibliophile, I research which books I allow to intruded upon my precious allotment of time, so I am seldom displeased with my choice of reading, be it for pleasure or research. But there are times when all that preparation and forethought does not work out and I find myself ensconced inside a bad read. What do I do? I sadly shake my head, offer a nod of apology to the author, who I know firsthand toiled at the keyboard for his or her art and passion, and put the book aside. Why?

"Because life's too short to read bad books."

~ Mike Foster

In fact, when you think about the amount of time we are allowed to spend on this planet, alive, existing, doing that thing called living our lives, it is but a mere dust mote of time. Time that should not be wasted. Why?

Because life's too short...to not do all the things you need and want to do to be all that you must to fulfill your time on earth.

Not to say that we shouldn't kick back, stop and smell the flowers, chill out with friends and family doing nothing but enjoying the moment. Of course not; all of the above are necessities in living one's life completely, to its fullest. Balancing one's priorities with hobbies, relaxation, enjoyment, and all those things in between is part of the challenge of daily existence.

My point today is not to waste your time, or life, by doing anything that does not make you happy, more enriched, better, smarter, healthier, wealthier, more spiritual...fulfilled. Why?

Because life's too short to...(fill in the blank).

If you hate your job, leave it. When I talk to people who appear miserable with their jobs, I tell them that I feel sorry for them that they have miserable lives. They look at me, shocked, and say that their life is not miserable, only their jobs. To that I say to them:

"If you hate your job you in essence hate your life. Change it."

And not just a career that is making you unhappy, but any other aspect of your life. If you don't like where you live, or with whom you live, think about it. That is a major part of your days, your time on earth. If it is not the situation that you want, you need to look into the whys and hows and ways to remedy that situation. Easier said than done, yes, but ignoring a problem is not fixing it.

And ignoring our life is, well, a waste of a life. After all, it's your life, your time on earth, and the last thing anyone wants to do in their golden years is to look back ruefully at a life unfulfilled, wasted, and not the one that you envisioned living. Think about it.

Life's too short to…

Do anything that you should not be doing that gets in the way of living your life to its fullest, every day in every way, 365.

I'd love to hear your comments on some of the things that you feel are a waste of your life…and how you are trying to change them, and your life, for the better.

peace,

Mike

TO ERR IS HUMAN...

You know the rest of that saying, right?

"To err is human, to forgive divine."

I like to take that admirable adage a few steps further and say that admitting one's mistakes, owning up to a shortcoming or just one bad moment is equally, if not more, important than forgiveness.

We all screw up, hence the above quote—we are all human beings so we are expected, at times, to do things poorly, say things in anger, misinterpret an emotion, or just plain boot a grounder at Fenway Park.

Mike's keys to dealing with being human:

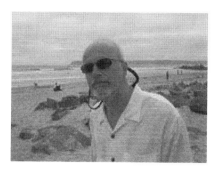

- Cut yourself some slack—if you were a robot then all your problems would be solved with a new microchip or a good reprogramming.

- Cut others even more slack—if we all have to jump in the pool and splash around in the muck, you do too! Forgiveness is a two-way street.

- When in doubt send flowers—or at least send love. Some people take longer to heal, are more sensitive, need time to get over whatever you did to make them so upset with you.

- Learn from it—what's the sense of being in the doghouse, groveling your way out, mending that fence you almost destroyed, if you just go back and do it again? Messing up can build more character than succeeding, at times.

I'm not saying that you should not always strive to do your best, just don't take yourself too seriously. Perfectionists are some of the most miserable people on the planet. While, when you think about it, children are some of the happiest. Why do you think that is? Kids are always messing up, making mistakes, doing something they shouldn't be doing. Yet most of them look at these childhood blunders as part of growing up, and learn from them. And youngsters are also some of the most forgiving creatures around, save for puppies.

"If you are not making mistakes, you are not trying, and if you are not trying you are not living."

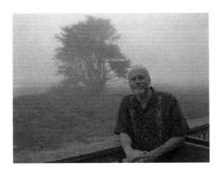

Sometimes life gets in the way of some of the things we want to accomplish. There's nothing you can do about it—it's life! Except react as best you can. Sadly, sometimes we react in the worst possible way. When that happens, make the best of it:

- Learn from it

- Improve self

- Value the experience

- Earn back trust

- Love

- Inspire

- Forgive

- Enjoy

365

Every day in every way.

peace,

Mike

NEAR DEATH—MORE LIFE!

We all saw it, that amazing photo of the plane that went down in the

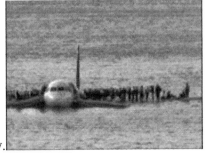

Hudson the other day. All those lucky
people standing on the wings of US Airways flight 1549 as it slowly sank
into the icy water. Survivors with nothing more than damp shoes and socks
as a reminder of what could have been as ferryboats arrived to motor them
back to dry land. The pilot, expertly and swiftly reacting to a flock of geese
that took out not one but both engines, a reluctant hero. A horrible disaster
averted. Elation, rather than tragedy, painting the faces of not only those
who survived and their relieved families, but a recharged country, and
world, desperately in need of some good news for a change.

I think I speak for many of you out there when I say that watching your life
flash before your eyes, or vicariously viewing it through the eyes of those
survivors of that doomed flight, reinvigorates your life. It makes you
grateful, true, but also reminds us of the precariousness of life, the gift that
we are given every day that allows us to breathe, to live. It also, no doubt,
forces us to take accountability for our actions, our lives—are we living our
lives, every day, the best we can? And why does it-all-too-often take a near-
death experience for us to embrace this precious and fragile thing called
life?

Have you ever had a near-death experience? I have; a few of them.

Besides feeling relieved and elated, frightened and thankful, what else can
we learn from near-death experiences? The answer, as always, can be found
at livelife365.

LIVE LIFE!
EVERY DAY,
EVERY WAY.

Life should never be taken for granted, and certainly never wasted. But so many of us, myself, at times, included, do just that. We need a near-death, or more optimistically put, a miracle, to awaken inside us what most of us

already know. Why is that? I'm not sure, but I feel that sometimes life, with its repetition and routine, its nightly news forecasts of financial doom, war, uncertainty, and sadness, wears us down. To the point of forgetting how wonderful life actually is. And while most of us try to look at the more positive sides of life, we still, more times than we like to admit, forget to greet each day as an opportunity to do something great, practicing patience and kindness, being positive and enterprising, and embracing the gift that has been bestowed upon us. Because, like it or not, we are not going to get out of this alive.

Bringing us back to that miraculous landing on the Hudson that could have started this New Year with tragedy, rather than hope. And reminding us how lucky we are.

Now, what are you going to do about it?

Huh?

We just got a fantastic wake-up call. Well, time to wake up, right?

Right. Wake up and not only smell the coffee (or green tea), but embrace this miracle called life every day. To its fullest. By being the best we can be and doing all that we can to live our lives 365.

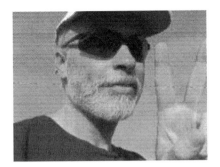

peace,

Mike

DO YOU BELIEVE?

A few weeks ago, I had the honor of participating in my brother's wedding. The celebration was thrown together in a short period of time due to medical circumstances of which I will not elaborate. Let me just say that in little more than a month's time, my brother and his amazing bride created a memorable, spectacular, and emotional event that had the look and feel of years of planning.

But something else occurred that day, an event that borders on the otherworldly, hints at Divine Intervention, and whispers of miracle.

Now do I have your attention?

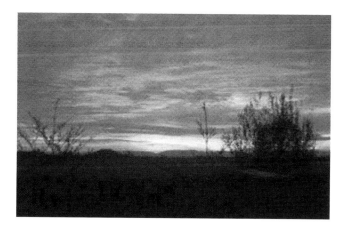

My father was taken from our family way too early—gone from this earth in his mid-50's, the victim of heavy cigarette and alcohol addictions that left him gasping for breath through emphysema-ravaged lungs. His death changed my life. It was not long after he died that I took control of my own self-destructive habits and turned my life around. But this post is not about my life, it is about my father…and how he may have attended my brother's wedding.

After days of worrying about the possibility of rain ruining things, the day turned out to be spectacular—a vital factor for an outdoor wedding. The venue was stunning: one of the oldest hotels on a scenic island in the littlest state in the Union. With the shimmering bay and majestic bridge as a backdrop, the wedding party stood excited and ready before hundreds of well-wishers. Dark clouds rolled in, not to dampen the spirit of the day, but instead arrived to offer a protective canopy of shade from the harsh sun.

I was relaxed, content, happy to be standing beside my brother, enjoying the ceremony, offering an occasional glance at family and friends in the crowd. Everything was going well, everything was normal…when overhead I heard the drone of an engine, barely noticeable at first, then gradually building in intensity. Being on public display, I didn't want to disrupt the ceremony with any overt actions or gestures, but as the noise built and it became obvious what was causing it—a jet, seemingly from out of nowhere, buzzing the quietude—I couldn't help myself.

I surreptitiously canted my head and caught sight of the plane as it burst through a gray cloud and soared into a sea of blue, the sun glinting off one wing, which seemed to tilt just as my eyes made contact with it.

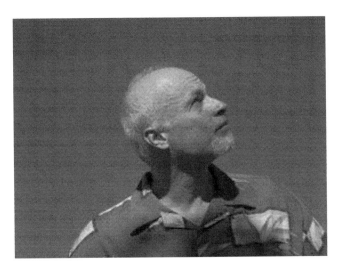

As the jet motored across the partially cloudy sky, and the words of the wedding ceremony sang in my ears, an almost surreal sensation overcame me—Dad! That was my father in that jet plane! A sad and satisfied smile tugged at the corners of my mouth and, as the plane's engines sounds began to fade into the background, I returned my focus and attention back to the wedding.

My father flew jets in the Navy. He was one of those brave pilots who land on aircraft carriers in the middle of the ocean. When he left the service, he flew small prop planes. (One of my biggest childhood thrills was going up in one of those planes and my dad allowing me to "co-pilot" the aircraft.)

A few hours into the wedding reception, I ran into my uncle, my father's brother. He asked if I had noticed the jet flying over during the ceremony. In a flash, the image of that plane, and all those strange sensations associated with its sudden appearance during the ceremony, came rushing back to me. I told my uncle I had seen it, why?

"I thought of your father," he said. "In fact, I thought it *was* your father."

An eerie chill trilled my flesh.

"So did I," I told him.

We looked at each other, both of us realizing the absurdity of our wishful thinking, while sharing a secret smile of hope and dreams and faith that perhaps it was not so far-fetched after all.

"Because," my uncle added, "this is not a normal flyover route, you know. And there was no air traffic before the wedding and none since that jet. Strange, huh?"

You don't know the half of it.

Much later on that long and happy day, in the wee hours of the morning, I repeated to my brother my conversation with our uncle, as well as my own observations about that lone jet. He said he'd not noticed the jet, but was elated to think that it could have been dad. In fact, he said he had no doubt that it must have been our father. (Of course, he had been partying a bit.) Then he added this bombshell: his new bride's father (also no longer of this world) also flew jets! Not only was our dad in that ethereal plane, but perhaps her father was, too.

As my brother rushed off, jubilation and awe painting his over-celebrated face, to share this revelation with this new bride, I sat back and reflected on the day...on that moment.

Was it real?

Did it happen?

Was it only a jet gliding overhead, oblivious to the events below?

Or was it…?

Because, after all, what is faith but the belief in something we are unable to prove exists.

Think about it.

peace,

Mike

PERSONAL DEVELOPMENT
III. BALANCE

10 THINGS I MUST DO EVERY DAY

Livelife365 is all about doing. Doing something positive every day. Something healthy. Spiritual. Exercising your body, yes, but also your mind. And your spirit. When I created livelife365 I wanted to share with as many people as possible helpful tips and successful programs that I have developed through the years, using videos and blog posts, like this one. Most of the successes that I talk and write about are things that I do every single day. Maybe that's why this site is called livelife365.

What are some of the things—positive, useful, invigorating, creative, important, worthwhile, fun, healthy, entertaining, fulfilling—things that you do each day?

TEN THINGS I MUST DO EVERY DAY

1. Exercise. Break a sweat. Do something physical, be it just taking a walk or lifting weights and riding my stationary bike. Even if you detest working out you can still get plenty of exercise chasing your kids around the yard, doing housework, washing the car, walking to the mailbox, or rolling around in bed with your significant other.

2. Enjoy the great outdoors. You don't have to live in the mountains or by a beach to appreciate the natural wonder and beauty of the earth. I go outside as often as possible during the day. Summertime is easier, but I still see many folks walk from house to car to work to car to house without stopping to smell the flowers or bask in the splendor. Taking a walk is an excellent way to get your exercise in while also listening to the birds. Plus the sun offers vitamin D, an essential necessity.

3. Meditate. I meditate every morning. My goal is at least thirty minutes of just sitting in a quiet room, eyes relaxed, sometimes closed, most times half-closed, clearing the clutter from my brain, listening to the sounds around me other than the thoughts in my head. It's easier than you may think, and well worth a few minutes of your day.

4. Drink green tea. I used to be a soda junkie, drank over five cans of Diet Coke a day. Not only is all that caffeine bad for you, but the other junk they put in soda can remove corrosion from a carburetor…imagine what it does to your stomach. When I gave up soda several years ago I started drinking green tea, and have never looked back. Green tea tastes great, is loaded with antioxidant and *polyphenols,* which help the immune system and protect against cancer and heart disease. Green tea also settles your stomach, not upsets is like with soda, and it can help you lose weight, lower your cholesterol, and even fight tooth decay. Get the idea I dig green tea? You should too.

5. Laugh. Sounds simple, sounds easy, sounds, well, rather silly to put on my list, but you'd be amazed how many people don't laugh enough—especially at themselves. Having a sense of humor goes a long way toward helping heal whatever ails you. And it's fun!

6. Eat healthy. Easier said than done for way too many people, but enjoying a healthy diet of fresh veggies and fruit, whole grains, beans and legumes, low in bad fats and high in fiber is the fuel that makes me who I am. The best part, besides being good for you and aiding in helping you live a longer, happier, healthier life, is all these healthy foods taste amazing. Don't let those fast food commercials fool you. A farm fresh tomato on whole wheat is one of the tastiest things you can eat…my mouth is watering already.

7. Pursue my hobbies. I play my guitar every day—sing, write music, just enjoying the sound. That's one of my hobbies, I have many more: gardening, landscaping, writing, videography, book collecting. We work, we rest, we enjoy time with family and friends, we eat and go to bed. In between you must try to find the time to do something for yourself—hobbies will get you to the place you need to be.

8. Read. Speaking of hobbies, I have had a voracious appetite for books ever since I can remember. I love to read. I read every single day of my life. I usually have several books going at one time—fiction, non-fiction, humorous, historical. I also devour newspapers and magazines…not to mention spending way too many hours of my life at my day job, reading endless tomes there. Reading is my great escape as well as my daily bread.

9. Think positive thoughts. I am a firm believer that no matter how bad things get—and life WILL deal you bad stuff—you have to remain positive. You have that power, something only you can control. Even if I'm having a particularly dreadful day for reasons that only astrologers and weathermen can explain, I still try to find something positive inside the gloom. And more often than not my sour mood turns better, and I shake my head and wonder why I was so down in the first place. Again, life is going to get all of us at times, but we have the power to fight back with positivity.

10. Floss. Every day. Besides brushing after every meal, I floss every night before bedtime. We only get one set of choppers so we have to take good care of them. Flossing is actually good for your heart, as well as reaching all those nooks and crannies inside your maw that your toothbrush cannot. Like my oral hygienist likes to say, *"You only have to floss the teeth you want to keep."*

I'm sure there are a few more things I do each day that didn't make my top ten list, but it's a good list. For me. What about you? We all have certain things that we need to do every day to live the life we want and need—these are some of mine. Hope your list is as healthy and happy and as fulfilling as mine is.

peace,

Mike

THE TRIAD OF BALANCE

When you get right down to it, life is a balancing act. We constantly strive to balance everything—Work and play. Self time and time spent with our significant others, children, other family members and friends. Serious, reflective moments (like this post) balanced against silly, goofy ones. Whether we are attempting to find the time to start or maintain an exercise program, or just steal an extra hour from our week to sink into a favorite chair and catch up on that novel we've been dying to read, the need for balance in our lives is a daily, often hourly, task.

But what about the need for balance inside each of us? What are you talking about, huh, Mike?

Triad of Balance.

Before we can find the time to balance our hectic lives, or begin to understand how to approach doing so, we need to balance our selves.

There are three parts of each of us that I feel need to be individually balanced—**Mind. Body. Spirit.** And then they need to be balanced together.

Let's start with the **Mind,** because once we have our head on straight, the rest falls into place nicely. The brain needs to be fed. There are lots of things that our mind absorbs each second—this post, for instance. The good thing is: we can, most of the time, choose what we ingest mentally. I suggest we feed our mind nothing but the good stuff, by that I mean: read more, watch TV less—or watch TV programs that add interesting, informative, positive data to our brain. That goes for what we read too—read fiction, sure, but a variety of it. Also everything else that stretches our limitations, help to learn new things, or add more positive, thought provoking images to our brain. Focus on the good in the world, while acknowledging the not so good, but remaining positive throughout. The more positive, intelligent, happy, helpful, kind, intriguing, beautiful (add your own positive word here) thoughts we incorporate into our brain every day, the healthier, happier, and more balanced we will become.

We also need to exercise our **Mind**. Just like muscles that do not stay active, an inactive brain will become flabby, less sharp. Work both sides of the brain: do puzzles (I love crosswords; do one a day), challenge yourself by learning a musical instrument, or joining a group like Toastmasters or by enrolling in a night college course.

Let's move from the **Mind** for now and focus on the **Body**. If we need to feed our brain with good, healthy data, you can probably guess what I'm going to say next, right? Remember that old expression? You are what you eat. What we eat and the amounts are vital in maintaining our body's balance. Eat healthy, nutritious foods and our bodies will respond in kind. Keep portion size down, and our body will not only be the right size, but it will help reduce some of the risks of heart disease (the number one killer in America), cancer, diabetes, hypertension, gastrointestinal problems, and any number of other maladies. Add to that healthy diet a sensible exercise program, and our body is going to love us. Speaking of love, let's add that to the list of things the brain should focus on each day.

We also need to keep the **Body** (and **Mind** and **Spirit**) free from negative intruders—tobacco, excessive alcohol, and dangerous drugs.

Treat your **Body** like the temple it is and you will feel great, live longer, and get yourself that much closer to being balanced.

Now the **Spirit**. Spirituality means different things to different people, but with one common bond—the act of doing something positive that fulfills us. And just like with the **Mind** and **Body**, our **Spirit** needs to be fed and exercised daily.

Feed your soul with happy, healthy, helpful thoughts, daily, then expand outward—share a funny joke with friends, call your mother or father on the phone just to say hello, offer a random act of kindness to a stranger, (leave a nice comment on someone's blog post). On a larger scale, we can do volunteer work, give to charity (money or time), join groups or forums with like-minded people practicing spiritual giving. And, of course, worship our higher power at our place of worship, or at home.

Now the hard part—balancing all three: **Mind, Body**, and **Spirit**.

There are times, too rare, when I have had my **Triad of Balance** in harmony, when I have felt mentally healthy and happy, physically strong and active, and spiritually fulfilled and content. But more often than not, one, or sometimes two, of the three need work. And when even one of the three is off, the result is: I am out of balance. Put another way: I am not complete, not the person I know I can be.

The ultimate goal, for me at least, is to have all three—**Mind, Body**, and **Spirit**—in balance all the time. While that is often a mighty challenge, it is one that, when attained, makes me the best person I can be, and well worth the effort.

Remember, as flawed human beings all we can do is try. Work at everything I've discussed here, each and every day, and good things are bound to happen.

peace,

Mike

FINDING THE TIME

When was the last time you were bored? The last time you had a handful of precious, unaccounted for moments with which you had absolutely nothing planned to do? A gap of time when all of your tasks and chores and obligations were, miraculously, completed, finito, no longer looming over your head like your father at your bedroom door giving you the stink eye on a Saturday morning while the front lawn beckons to be mowed.

Me? I consider myself very lucky to never seem to have a dull day, strewn with large chunks of nothing-to-do time, peppered with bouts of ennui and salted with hours of endless emptiness. On the other hand, I sometimes find myself craving the simpler things in life, like lounging with a cold beverage by the ocean with no decision more pressing than where, oh, where will we dine tonight? Or holed up in a secluded cabin in the middle of nowhere with a hundred books I've been putting off and dying to read. But, alas, those scenarios only exist in my fantasy dreams and a few weeks a year during my much needed and very much appreciated vacation time.

Back to reality. I like to keep busy; enjoy it, actually. But it goes beyond that. You could say that I am driven to succeed, to accomplish as much as I can in the short amount of time we have on this earth. And while that's a good thing, it can present challenges. Of course, keeping ones balance amidst all the madness is a must, but finding the time to do all that needs to be done is equally, if not more, important.

"It is a vital necessity to do all the things that you have to do to be able to achieve all the things that you need to do."

--Mike Foster

I love a life filled with activity, of as many positive endeavors you can shake a stick at, especially those that enhance, improve, grow, shape, and drive you as a person. The key is finding the time to do as much of all this good stuff as humanly possible. Here are some tips:

- prioritize…then prioritize again
- multitask
- eliminate "empty" activities
- turn that boob tube off!
- learn to juggle
- don't bite off more than you can chew
- practice patience
- at the end of the day, pat yourself on the back and…
- …write a new to-do list
- do it all over again

Remember, it's good to be busy, but also just as important to find the balance to do other things unrelated to deadlines and pressures, tasks and chores, goals and obligations. I understand the importance of living a balanced life, but also the necessity of living a fulfilled one. The key is:

FINDING THE TIME

peace,

Mike

BALANCE. HAVE YOU CHECKED YOURS LATELY?

Trick question? Are we talking mentally, physically, or spiritually? Actually, I'm talking about all three. Right now, for instance, I am struggling to find a nice balance between an increased workload and the need to relax. Time, it seems, is swallowed up by this blog and my vlog, my full-time job (you know, the one that pays the bills), and all the little things that go on in between the three. I cannot recall a day or hour lately when I felt bored. And that's a good thing, for the most part. I am a firm believer that human beings are happiest when they are busy, driven, leading a purposeful life. But we still need balance.

What's the old saying? All work and no play makes Jack a dull boy? Well, I don't know how dull I've been of late, but I sure am beat. More to the point: I am out of balance. I looked in the mirror the other day and almost didn't recognize myself. Gazing back at me was this sunken-cheeked guy, with five days of growth on his face, huge dark circles rimming his eyes. But beneath that haggard looking facade I noted a hint of a satisfied smirk, a contented grin. Yet, still, I was not complete, whole. Balanced.

I have a program, which I am in the process of turning into a book, called "Triad of Balance." What this is (the short version) is working every day to get yourself in balance. Get your triad in balance. The triad being: Mind. Body. Soul. All the while, as you strive for balance in each area (Intellectually, Physically, Spiritually), the ultimate goal is to then get those three in balance with each other. I will touch more on these principles in coming blogs. In the meantime, if you can't wait (the book will not be out for several months), I have a video about this on my website that goes into more detail than I will in this entry.

Now, back to why I am out of balance right now. By working too many hours, I have been neglecting to work on other aspects of my life. Other areas that, if ignored too long, will rise up and bite you. It is vital to; first, understand what your mind, body, and spirit need daily to be complete. And then essential that you make yourself do these things. I know that I need to work out almost every day. That I need a certain amount of sleep. That, even though I love the work that I do every day, I also need to feed the other parts of my brain: reading for pleasure, relaxing and talking with my wife, walking outside, dining out, or just sitting in front of the TV, watching a funny sitcom, doing a crossword puzzle. Simple tasks, not as important, it seems, than working at earning a living. But vital for your balance. Essential. Any of this sound familiar to you?

I just briefly touched on the edges of the importance of living a balanced life and offered up a few remedies. Remember, the key is your understanding of what YOU need in your daily existence to make you whole. And don't forget your Triad: Mind. Body. Soul. Because, if even one of the Big Three is out of whack, you will be out of whack. Even if you are balanced intellectually and physically, but lacking balance spiritually, you will not be complete. Think about it. One step at a time. One area at a time. Then work on getting all three balanced. The good news? The more conscious you are of your needs, and the more you strive to attain them, the closer you will be to getting where it is you need to be. And even if some days you are slightly off, a little unbalanced in one area, by understanding what you need to do to get back on track you are that much better off. As for me, I vow to work less and spend more time relaxing with my lovely wife. Maybe take a scenic walk with her through one of the many wonderful parks we have here in town. In between that, think I will park it on the couch with a pile of magazines and newspapers, put the Red Sox on the tube, sip some green tea, and, if all goes well, nod off and catch up on some sleep.

Balance. Have you checked yours lately?

peace,

Mike

ENTERTAINMENT

I. HUMOR

THE SIGNIFICANCE OF LAUGHTER

Such a serious title for something as benign as laughter. Yes, it is, but for a reason. The need to laugh, to find humor in things sometimes unfunny, to chuckle, giggle, guffaw, shriek, snort, or titter, may be one of the best remedies for what ails you.

Humor is serious business. Huh? That's right. We need to laugh just as much as we need to eat or sleep. Think about how you feel when deprived of your recommended nightly hours of sleep—not too good, right? How about when your stomach is reminding you that you have not eaten recently, or that you have and that it was not sitting well down there. Again, not a pleasant sensation. Same can be said about those who do not get enough laughter in their daily lives. Eat, drink, and be merry. Perhaps there was something to that ancient adage after all?

One of the reasons I created livelife365 (both my website and this blog) was to be able to reach as many people as possible, sharing with them all the myriad ideals and ideas, videos and music, helpful programs and proven theories that I have amassed over the years. But the best part is that I not only can help others lose weight or eat right, gain self-esteem or proper balance, but that I can entertain them. Make them laugh. It's no accident that livelife365 offers more than most blogs or websites, a more diverse menu of entrees. I want to be able to help and teach, council and coach, share and learn, yes, but I also get a great deal of satisfaction when I put a smile on someone's face.

I have been asked,"Mike, how can you be treated seriously as a self-help guru when you are constantly acting like a goofball in some of your videos?" My response to that is: If I made you laugh, then it was worth it. Livelife365 is all about life, and the importance of living your life each day to its fullest. Yes, adhering to a healthy lifestyle is vital, as is proper mental focus and self-development. But all that and not enough joy, humor or laughter in your life is an incomplete life. An unfulfilled life.

One of my favorite programs is called Triad of Balance. This is about getting your mind, body, and spirit in balance as one, after working on balancing each one individually. It is easier said than done, but finding daily laughter in your life will help your balance in each area—Mind; Body; Spirit. That, in a nutshell, should underscore the importance of laughter. The significance of finding humor every day.

Good luck, here's to a hearty chuckle today, hopefully much more than one. If you need help, visit my website and mouse over LAUGH. There you will discover dozens of, most of the time, funny videos that should do the trick. If not, let me know what tickles your funny bone and I will do my best to put a smile on your face.

peace,

Mike

WHEN IN DOUBT, YANK 'EM OUT!

Is there anything more painful than a toothache?

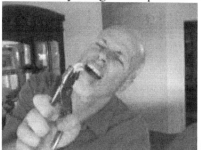 Okay, maybe a gunshot wound, but, thankfully, having never experienced being shot I can't really make a valid comparison. Childbirth? Being of the wrong gender, I am legally not allowed to comment. How about having an angry ex-(anyone) rearing back and kicking you squarely in the lower region naughty parts? Having **HAD** experience with that, I can honestly say that, while having your family jewels rearranged is quite painful, a prolonged toothache is worse. How much worse? Bad enough to pay someone (a large chunk of cash) to knock you out under anesthesia and then take a sharp carving implement and have at the insides of your mouth.

It all started with a little ache in the lower left side of my mouth. Being an avid tooth-brusher and compulsive flosser, as well as a regular dental checkup kind of guy, I figured the pain would go away, like one hopes an annoying neighbor will. Sadly, that is the wrong strategy to use for both toothaches and neighbors, so I paid a visit to my dentist. He probed and poked, x-rayed and consulted until he reached suitable recompense, then announced that I had a fractured tooth and that I should…

"Yes, yes?" I said, nodding hopefully, knowing that relief was just a few magical dental moves away.

"Wait," my (not usually sadistic) dentist said.

"Huh?" said I.

"It's fractured. Can't fill it, can't extract it, so just wait until…"

"Yes? Until…?"

"Until it either fractures some more or you need a root canal."

After one more "huh?" and a few "what the…?'s", my dentist smiled, nodded, and left me with drool on my chin and a still sensitive tooth in need of…what?

Patience.

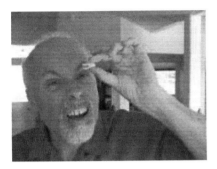

So I waited, continued to eat my almonds and enjoy my dietary life as usual, while favoring that fractured side of my mouth. This went on for months and months, until…

AAARRRGGGOOOOOOOOCCCHHHHH!

The fracture fractured some more, creating enough pain to motivate me to make another visit to my dentist, who, after more adequate probing and x-raying to satisfy his curiosity and my deductible, announced:

"Looks like you may need a root canal."

Through a mouthful of fingers, cotton, and that annoying little sucking machine, I said, ***"Warrgllehuhphmmm?"***

My dentist smiled, nodded, added up my bill and decided to take one more x-ray, then shuffled me off to another practitioner of dental maneuvers: an endodontist, who specialized, I was told, in root canals, more probing, vague announcements, and, of course, additional x-ray taking. The biggest difference I noticed was that the endodontist charges more and it takes longer to get an appointment. But if you tell them that you are in extreme pain, they will smile, recheck their appointment book, then tell you that whining won't make the pain go away so take some Advil and practice…

Patience.

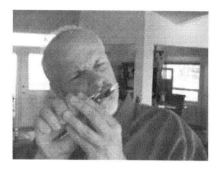

And that's what I did, finally getting the pleasure of having a higher paid sadist probe my fractured tooth, while feeling the stirring of another tooth announce its painful presence on the other side of my mouth. So I said:

"What the heck, doc, it's only money, right? Take a look at that other guy while you're at it."

My endodontist nodded, grunted, probed, ordered and received additional x-rays, probed some more then pondered and professed:

"You need two root canals. How much money do you have?"

My mouth stuffed with the expensive hands of a specialist, cotton, a dental assistant, and that annoying little sucky thing that sometimes gets stuck in the back of your throat, making you want to vomit and choke at the same

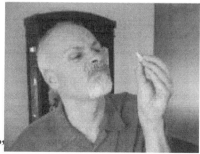

time, I said, ***"Whadrrrgfhrrfertwwwooo?"***

My sadistic little endodontist nodded, smiled, and left the room to order more x-rays. Leaving me to, you guessed it, practice…

Patience.

Finally the day arrived when I had my root canal exploratory exam that would let me know if I could save the fractured tooth, have the root canal, then be able to have a crown installed. The crown, of course, would be done by yet another dental practitioner and cost several arms, a leg, and the promise of donating various organs to science and x-ray development costs.

His hands deep inside my mouth, which was benumbed by enough Novocain to curtail the charge of a rabid rhinoceros, my endodontist announced:

"Tsk, tsk, bad news. Fracture is too deep, no root canal, have to have it extracted. I must leave now because you are no longer a viable money stream, but before you go let's take a few more x-rays just to be sure."

With that he left, leaving me with a numb face, two still very throbbing teeth, and an appointment with another dental professional.

While all this was going on, over the course of several months, I favored one side of my mouth over the other, effectively adding additional stress to that side, effectively causing the tooth that wasn't yet fractured

to **SPLIT IN HALF!!** This caused me enormous pain, and more trips to dental professionals, along with, you guessed it:

MORE X-RAYS!!

Finally leading me to this past Friday, where, after all three geniuses of the dental community, otherwise known as the Mike Foster Dental Retirement Fund Group, decided it was best that I had both fractured and root-befouled teeth extracted.

I, of course, had to find yet another dental practitioner, who, of course, took several more x-rays, and then, naturally, checked the balance of my dental coverage to make sure he charged enough, and then, thankfully, mercifully, at long last:

REMOVED MY TWO THROBBING TEETH!

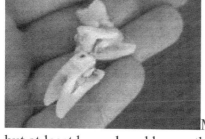Making my pain not necessarily go away, but at least be replaced by another pain, a healing, slightly bloody, cheek-puffing pain that while still nowhere near where I want to be pain-wise, at least was better than what I had been feeling for the past half-year.

The good news is I am feeling better every day, those two annoying teeth are gone (along with several painful extractions from my wallet and checking accounts), and I am well on my way to the road to recovery.

Hmmm, maybe just one more x-ray?

peace,

Mike

MY MOM IS "SEEING" THE GUY WHO USED TO STEAL MY BALLS

I just got off the phone with my mom. She lives Back East. She is a recent widow. This past December, my stepfather passed away, and my mom now occupies their large home by herself. While still grieving, she is determined to move on with her life, to persevere, to live life 365, like my website suggests. Little did I know how determined she was!

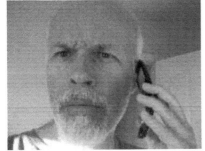

Like I said, I just hung up the phone (or, in this age of flip-open cell phones: I snapped it closed and slipped it back into my pocket) after experiencing a rather odd conversation with my mother. Now, more often than not, a conversation with my mom borders on oddness, meanders around the strange, and all too frequently is laced with nonsensical utterances. This one was no exception, except she also added that, a mere three months since the passing of my stepfather, she was *"seeing"* someone. Not *"dating"* someone. According to those seventy-something romantics, *"seeing"* is strictly dining and watching a movie together. While *"dating"* is something that my fifty-something brain cannot, will not, and refuses to wrap itself around. The bizarre conversation went something like this:

MIKE: *Hi, Ma, how are you holding up?*

MOM: Oh, fine, just fine…doing better.

MIKE: *That's great. So, what's new?*

MOM: Oh, you know, nothing much. (sounds of fork and knife against dishes and food being masticated)

MIKE: *Same here. What are you doing, eating? Want me to call back?*

MOM: Oh, no, it's okay. (whispering sounds away from the phone)

MIKE: *Is someone there?*

MOM: Huh? (giggle)

MIKE: *Ma?*

MOM: I'm here... (away from the phone): No, let me get that, Dave (not his real name)

MIKE: *Dave?*

MOM: Oh, he's trying to put the dishes away.

MIKE: *Huh?*

MOM: Huh? (giggle, sounds of dishes clattering, more chewing sounds, and something that may or may not have been a belch)

MIKE: *Huh?*

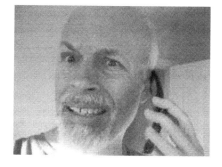

MOM: Michael?

MIKE: *Ma? What's going on?*

MOM: Oh, you remember Dave? From the neighborhood?

MIKE: *Dave? What's he doing there?*

MOM: (away from the phone): Michael says "hi."

MIKE: *Ma?*

On and on it went like that, only it got worse, took stranger and weirder turns until my head was spinning like a gyro. Through my dizziness, I finally found the fortitude to say goodbye and hang up. After several minutes of mental Ping-Pong, I debated having my first drink of real alcohol since 1993.

You see, besides my shock at discovering my mom was *"seeing"* someone less than three months after my stepfather went off to meet his Maker, I was taken aback by her choice of gentleman callers. Not that there is anything wrong with Dave (not his real name); actually, Dave is a great guy. Now. But back in the day, when I was a wild child, a hyperactive menace, an energy-driven sports junkie, I kicked, tossed, hurled, belted, flipped, flew, flung, booted, upchucked, and projectile-vomited every known object of recreational activity—baseball, bat, glove, Frisbee, tennis ball, football, badminton racket, golf club, shuttlecock, and kickball—into our neighbor's fenced-in backyard…into our neighbor Dave's (not his real name) yard. And do you know what Dave did? *Hmmm?*

HE KEPT THEM! ALL OF THEM! EVERY SINGLE ONE OF THEM!

Today, as a moderately mature adult, I can certainly understand where Dave (still not his real name) was coming from. Who would want some snot-nosed brat shucking and shoveling every ball or sports equipment known to man into his backyard? Not me—now! And certainly not Dave, then!

But as a kid, an athletic kid who adored sports and wanted nothing more than to run wild in his yard playing make-believe Red Sox games in which he was at bat in the bottom of the ninth with the winning runs on base, I was devastated. And out a lot of balls. But I got better, got over it, moved on, actually forgot about it as the decades came and went and the balls of my youthful dreams evolved into balls that, in the name of good taste, shall remain nameless.

And don't even get me started on the differences between *"seeing"* someone and actually *"dating"* them. To quote my mother:

"Oh, no, Michael, we're just friends, it will never come to that, and he understands that."

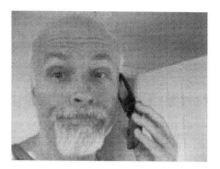

Me: *"Ma, come on, he's a man, even if he's in his seventies, he is a man and men would much rather 'date' someone that merely 'see' them."*

Leading me to this conclusion: what can ya do? I mean, she's a grown woman who knows, for the most part, what she's doing. If she wants to *"see"* the guy who used to steal my balls, then God bless her. It's better than *"dating"* the guy who used to steal my balls, I guess.

But do me one favor, huh, Ma? As this "seeing" eventually evolves into *"dating,"* and that morphs into something *I CANNOT EVEN BEGIN TO IMAGINE!*...can you do me one big favor? Huh?

Can you ask Dave (okay, really, not his real name...not even close) if he still has my balls? And if he does, can I have them back?

peace,

Mike

WALKING MY PET PEEVES

Most of my writing—and I certainly hope that you would agree with this—focuses on the positive, from my nutritional and fitness tips, to my motivational and inspirational messages—even my music and humorous stuff is created to not only entertain, but to educate, too.

Yet (and some close family members and lifelong friends may be inclined to debate this) I remain a human being, one with flaws, faults, foibles, and faux pas (and those are just the "F"s). I do not wear my Mike Foster-goofy-

grin-with-green-teacup face all the time, especially while I am in a car, either driving it or witnessing someone else manning the wheel.

Certain peccadilloes of human bizarre behavior seem to present themselves more frequently while scooting through traffic, many of these irk, irritate, infuriate, and raise my ire (and those are just the "I"s) to the point of adding them to my list of pet peeves.

Take, for example, the directional signal. This is one misused, seldom used, and overused instrument of driving that drives me nuts.

Scenario One: You're driving in a queue of traffic, approaching a left-turn-only lane, you:

a) drive into the lane, idle in traffic while waiting for the light to turn, then when the arrow turns green, and as you proceed to turn you put your left blinker on, effectively indicating to the other drivers that you are going to turn left…**IN A LEFT-TURN-ONLY LANE!!!**

b) Approach the intersection, start to weave into the left-turn-only lane, you stomp on your brakes, slow down to a maddening crawl, pull into your lane of choice…**THEN PUT ON YOUR DIRECTIONAL**, effectively indicating to the poor soul behind you that which he already knows.

c) You flip your directional indicator on several miles before your turn, click-click-clicking away in oblivious nirvana, then actually get into the left-turn-only lane, blinker blinking away like a manic tweaker, sitting in queue, click-click-clicking the obvious, then when the light turns green, continue through the intersection, your directional still snapping away as you proceed to make a left turn around the world.

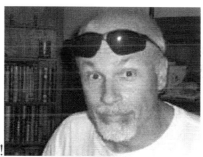

d) all of the above…are idiots!

As you can see I have a bit of a problem with the left-turn-only lane and the misuse of the directional signal. But my annoyance with blinkers does not stop there. How about the guy who swerves in front of you, sans blinker, slams on the brakes…**THEN PUTS HIS DIRECTIONAL ON!!** Why bother, buddy?

Then we have the fast lane versus the slow lane, or the left lane, what we used to call the passing lane back when I went to driver's education, and the right lane, the lane reserved for those who are related to snails.

Can someone explain to me why anyone drives in the left lane, the supposedly passing lane, and refuses to drive the speed limit—I'm talking about driving **BELOW** the speed limit?! Anyone?

While this pet peeve rankles, riles, and ruffles my feathers (that's right, those are just the "R"s), I also use it as a self-challenge in practicing patience…excellent time spent plotting diverse ways at torturing the slow-Joe creating his own personal parade in the high-speed lane. And then, after a month of driving behind this joker, I am finally able to pass, casting a stink-eye glance at the culprit…only to see that it is some harmless, kind-looking, elderly woman who bears such a striking resemblance to my mother my guilt overwhelms me to the point of almost driving into a tree.

Okay, I understand that most of us behave differently inside the protective, stereo-blasting, French fry-eating, cell phone-chatting, Facebook-updating safety of our own vehicles, but my last pet peeve so bothers, bugs, bewilders, and befuddles (uh-huh, just the "B"s) me I am almost at a loss for words…key word being "almost."

Smoking. Anyone or anything. Anywhere or anytime. I will never understand why anyone who has ever learned to read past the third-grade level would ever smoke a cigarette. Besides being the most rude, reprehensible, repulsive, and ridiculous (need I say that those are just the "R"s?) habit I can imagine, it has been proven to be so unhealthy for you that to ingest burning leaves of tobacco into your once clean lungs can only be the actions of a crazy person…or someone who needs my help.

Anyone who has ever shared an elevator car with someone who has just spent their fifteen minute break puffing away on a cancer stick understands what a preview of hell might be like.

Let's pretend smoking doesn't smell horrendous, or will kill you sooner rather than later, what about that dreaded smoker's cough? Working in an office, I am serenaded daily by the hacking wheeze of the chronic smoker's phlegm-filled foghorn bellowing from the mouths, throats, and, sadly, lungs of my clueless coworkers. Do I feel empathy and compassion? Yes. But I also feel sad and peeved, prompting me to take steps…like writing this, and praying and hoping that someday, very soon, these misdirected and weak individuals will get the help they need to live the life they surely desire.

So, next time I am driving to work, watching the click-click-clicking of a misguided directional signal in the car in front of me, who is also hogging the passing lane for reasons known only to he or she, and I am finally able to pass this "interesting" person, and I glance over and notice that he or she is puffing madly away on a cigarette, I will—gulp—nod, wave, smile, and continue on my way, ready to embrace my day, knowing that when in doubt:

TAKE YOUR PET PEEVE FOR A WALK!

You'll be glad you did.

peace,

Mike

ATTACK OF THE ROGUE PRETZEL

The other day, while reclining atop a hotel room bed, reading a magazine, I was attacked by a rogue pretzel. What, you may be asking yourself, was I doing eating pretzels on a hotel room bed? Well, I was attempting to embrace and enjoy a rare respite from the madness otherwise known as "my life," that's what. Happily trying to catch up on two months' worth of magazines, giddily avoiding my laptop, while shamelessly engaging in a rare caloric activity—namely shoveling empty calories of fun into my normally dietary-rigid mouth.

Perhaps that had something to do with this recalcitrant pretzel's sneak attack—my rustiness in the simple art of consuming snack foods. You see, I am a total health nut freak (recently I was slightly taken aback by a comment left on one of my posts that described me as a "health nut," until I sat back and thought about that word and realized, without a doubt, that, hey, I am a health nut! And that's a good thing). I rarely allow myself the pleasure of consuming snacks (like pretzels or potato chips—a HUGE snacking vice for me, by the way). But on occasion, and this was one of those (being on vacation), I cut myself a break and indulged in a salty treat…and it ended up not biting me in the backside, but stabbing me in the mouth.

Here's what happened: I was methodically cramming pretzel after pretzel into my seemingly insatiable maw, stick pretzels, you know the kind I mean, when one snapped in half, flipped up on to one end, and impaled itself into the roof of my mouth. Okay, maybe not impaled, but definitely jabbed, gouged, stabbed, shived, bayoneted, knifed, poked—name your bloody word! Because there was blood, lots of blood!

Needless to say, the elation of my pretzel pig-out was immediately and sadly cut short—as if the God of Nutrition had decided that he had seen enough, and reached his hand into my masticating mouth and manipulated a half-chewed pretzel into attention and to use as a weapon, thus putting an end to this empty-caloric nonsense.

Tossing the offending junk food bag into the corner of the hotel room, I hurried to the bathroom sink and rinsed and relieved my mouth of blood and all starchy remnants. I probed and stuffed balls of moistened tissue into my throbbing mouth until, after almost an hour's battle, the bleeding subsided, leaving me with a very sore palate, and zero desire to indulge in any salty, crunchy foods for the rest of this decade.

This harrowing brush with death (okay, maybe not my death, but at least the death of desire for a pretzel, once one of my few remaining guilty pleasures) left me pondering my lot in life, and reminded me of a similar incident, years ago, that involved our infamous lame duck resident of the White House. You remember, right? While eating pretzels and watching football on TV, good old George W. fainted and fell face first into oval office carpeting. Left with a bruised cheek and ego, he joked about it later, saying, "If my mother is listening, mother, I should have listened to you: Always chew your pretzels before you swallow."

Wow, me and the Prez. Some may be thinking: it couldn't have happened to two nicer guys…or something along those lines.

Better yet, the lesson I learned from all this is one I have been shouting from the rooftops for years and years, and that is:

JUNK FOOD KILLS!

…or at least attacks and maims.

peace,

Mike

IS IT JUST ME?

Picture this peaceful scenario:

I'm relaxing upon my sofa (or couch), in my serene living room, TV on, muted (as always), watching my beloved <u>Red Sox</u> as they battle for the pennant, my faithful laptop warming my lap (and transmitting God-knows-what variety of electrons and microwaves and unspeakable potential doom into my nether regions), enjoying the fruits of my (and my lovely wife's) labor. Ahh, nothing like living the American Drea--

**VRRRRRROOOOOOMMMMMM!!!!!
SCCCRRREEETCCCCHHHH!!!!!**

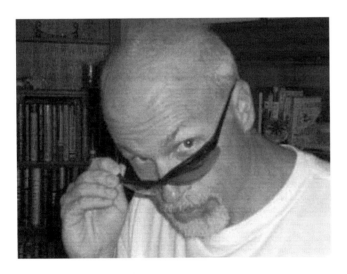

A car. Moving very fast. Speeding along my street. A street, by the way, that has a speed limit of 25 mph. A street, I might add, that stretches not much longer than the size of five house lots. (This being California, the Golden State, otherwise known as the state-with-postage-stamp-sized-lots, those lots are not large.) A street, if you will allow me to continue, that is situated between two stop signs, with my house smack-dab (I have never used this expression before, but it sounds so good here, doesn't it?)...ahem...smack-dab in the middle of those two stop signs.

My point being (and I **DO** have one), is that one (and when I say "one," I'm talking about dozens of [add your favorite expletive here]) would have to really, really **WANT** to seriously exceed the 25 mph speed limit to buzz so fast past my house--**AFTER STOPPING** (sometimes) at one stop sign, and then seeing (and knowing) that they need to stop again (rarely) at the next sign, a mere 100 feet (give or take; I've not measured it...yet) away.

IS IT JUST ME?

Or are these people (using the term very loosely) who are speeding through *my* neighborhood, to get to *their* neighborhood, not really people at all? But some as-yet-named (or discovered) species of animal (apologies to the Animal Kingdom) that feel it is okay to disrupt (and possibly endanger) my quietude (and solitude and, more importantly, my **RED SOX GAME**!) so they can practice their Indy maneuvers just so they don't miss a minute of *Wheel of Fortune*.

I am confused.

IS IT JUST ME?

I've talked about this before, and still have not come up with a solution that would keep me out of federal prison, so I shall move on to the next scenario.

You're sitting beside your lovely spouse, inside a swanky restaurant, maybe holding hands (or a shrimp, recently dipped in tangy cocktail sauce; me: a limp carrot stick), enjoying the ambiance. The background music is perfect, just loud enough so that you barely notice it, while not too much that it becomes a distraction. The service has been stellar, your beverages chilled just right and working their magic (hers, an appletini; mine: spring water...with a twist). Your salads arrive..."oh, yes, please, some fresh ground pepper would be wonderful, thank you--"

**"HELLO? OH, HEY, YA, NO, NOTHING. JUST HAVING DINNER.
GLAD YA CALLED. OH, YEAH? HAHAHAHAHAAAA! THAT'S**

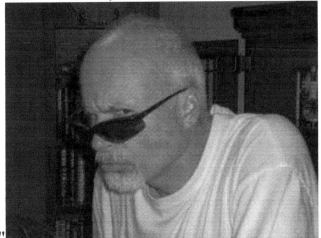

FUNNY!"

No, it's not.

IS IT JUST ME?

Or should people (call them what you want) who loudly yak on their cell
phones in pubic places (especially restaurants!) be:

a) tarred and feathered

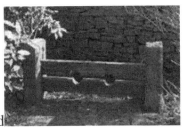

b) placed in <u>stocks</u> and be publicly humiliated

c) hog-tied and forced to watch as you delete the memory from their iPhone

d) dragged into the restaurant's kitchen and stuffed inside a:

    1) dishwasher
    2) deep fryer

   3) <u>Turducken</u>
   4) all of the above
Where was I?

Right, enjoying a very complicated, yet incredibly rewarding, daydream fantasy.

My point is:

CUT US ALL A BREAK!

The utter gall and deluded imagination involved in thinking that **ANYONE** other than your mother (and she's vacillating a bit, too, I might add), wants to listen to **YOUR** conversation while they are trying to enjoy a nice dining experience is beyond comprehensible, well past ludicrous, and speeding right over ridiculous.

IS IT JUST ME?

I mean, really? Is it--

Hold on, I gotta take this.

"YO? AH, NOTHING, JUST WRITING. NO, I'M IN MY CAR. SURE, BE RIGHT THERE. 'BYE."

**VRRRRRROOOOOOMMMMMM!!!!!
SCCCRRREEETCCCCHHHH!!!!!**

peace,

Mike

MY MOM MAKES ONE MEAN LASAGNA!

During my recent visit Back East to, among other things, attend my brother's wedding, I also stumbled upon a serendipitous epiphany of gourmet delectability.

Huh?

Big words (just showing off) that merely mean: **My Mom Makes One Mean Lasagna!**

One Mean *Vegetable* Lasagna, that is.

I grew up in a half-Italian household, by that I mean an Italian household. If you know Italians, then you understand that they have a tendency to dominate a room…or a home. Gastronomically speaking, this is a good thing! The funny thing is, my mom is not the Italian in the family; she's French. But by marrying an Italian man, she was bound by Sicilian tradition and old Francis Ford Coppola Films to learn, from a genuine Nana, how to make a tomato sauce from scratch. And also how to please the garlic- and olive oil-loving palate of a gentleman with a vowel at the end of this last name. The good news: she more than passed the test; she excelled.

Have I mentioned: My Mom Makes One Mean Lasagna!

So, when I informed my mother that I would be taking that big (not that big, actually) jumbo jet in the sky back to her neck of the woods to be among family and friends to celebrate her youngest child's nuptials, she naturally asked if she could cook something special for me. And I naturally requested her World Famous Lasagna…but with one catch.

Mike: Can you make me a *vegetable* lasagna?

Mom: Oh…I've never made one of those.

Mike: I know, that's why I'm asking you. No meatballs.

Mom: Oh…you used to love my meatballs.

Mike: Yes, Ma, I did, but I'm a vegetarian now. Remember?

Mom: Oh…right. You can't eat meatballs?

Mike: No meat, Ma. None. So, can you make a *meatless* lasagna?

Mom: Oh…I suppose. What kind of vegetables do you want?

Mike: Anything, surprise me.

Mom: Oh…

Mike: And no pork fat, please, in the sauce.

Mom: Oh…dear…what?

Mike: Mom?

Mom: Oh…but I always use pork fat.

Mike: Yes, I know. Can you use something else?

Mom: Oh…I suppose…

Mike: Mom?

Mom: Oh…

Mike: Mom?

Mom: Oh…

On and on it went until we agreed that olive oil would be a healthy and tasty alternative to the pork fat my mother usually adds to the saucepan in which to sauté the onions and garlic and whatever else she uses to start her World Famous Tomato Sauce.

During the weeks and days leading up to my trip Back East, my mother would call often, grilling me on my vegetable preferences.

Mike: Hello?

Mom: Michael, do you like mushrooms?

Mike: Huh?

Mom: For the lasagna.

Mike: Oh. Yeah, sure, love 'em.

Mom: How about your brother?

Mike: Huh?

Mom: Do you think he's allergic to them?

Mike: Huh?

Mom: Or his fiancée?

Mike: Huh?

Mom: How about eggplant?

Mike: Huh?

Mom: Cauliflower?

Mike: …

After numerous calls and some serious consideration of adding my mother's phone number to my "no-call" list, we settled on what will from this point on be known as "The Masterpiece."

I landed in my old state on a Monday and sat down to a small gathering of family and friends at mom's house on a Tuesday. My salivary glands the only part of my body not suffering from jet lag, I watched with utter amazement as my tiny mother removed from the oven a tray of vegetable lasagna, slightly larger than some of the carry-on luggage I saw my fellow air passengers unsuccessfully trying to cram into the overhead bin.

Heaped upon a plate before me was a wedge of lasagna, roughly the size of my head while wearing a large hat. I dug in. It melted in my mouth. The veggies were cooked just right; not too crunchy or too limp. And the tomato sauce was the best ever: savory and vibrant. Without the overpowering (sorry meat-eaters) presence of the meatballs and pork fat, I could taste more of the tomato and garlic, which also brought out the succulent olio of flavors from the broccoli, mushrooms, cauliflower, and eggplant.

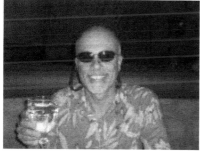

It was delicious!

It was "The Masterpiece."

When I stated that my mom made one mean lasagna, I wasn't kidding. Now I can emphatically add that:

My Mom Makes One Mean Vegetable Lasagna!

The moral of this story: For a healthier, tastier life, go veggie and hold the meatballs.

peace,

Mike

ENTERTAINMENT

II.   OPINION

CBS REPLACES CHARLIE SHEEN WITH A MONKEY!

I am sick and tired of hearing about Charlie Sheen. I barely watch TV, and certainly not the gossipy shows that live off the detritus of train wrecks like Carlos Estevez (his real name, by the way)—so for me to even be writing this means that this story is everywhere. And I do not like having it invade my space!

For those of you living under rocks or on some secluded island, Charlie Sheen is a television actor on a popular situation comedy who is too screwed up to show up for work. As a health and fitness guru, not to mention a self-help and personal development guy, I do have some empathy for the messed up Charlie's of the world—in fact, I would love to be the person who helps him and sets him on the path to enlightenment and recovery. But, alas, Charlie does not want help or feels he needs it. He is cool with who he is and how his behavior not only affects himself, but those around him. Still, I would be more than willing to work with him…if he asks.

Since I've not received any SOS flare from Chuck, I have instead decided to offer up a few suggestions on how CBS, the most-watched television network in these United States, should handle the sad case of Charlie Sheen.

REPLACE HIM WITH A MONKEY!!

Here are the bottom-line, no-nonsense facts: Charlie Sheen is just an actor, a very lucky actor who was able to take mediocre talent and transform it, along with an established family name, into an amazing career. He has been paid outrageous amounts of money for, basically, standing in front of a camera and reciting bad lines of dialogue that make millions laugh. Now, there's nothing wrong with making people laugh. I think finding humor in things throughout the day is a necessity in living one's life to its fullest, along with being one of the essences of living a healthy life.

But Sheen is just a guy who has a job that reaches millions…but **IT'S JUST A JOB! AND HE'S JUST A GUY! AND HE DID NOT SHOW UP FOR WORK BECAUSE OF SELFISH REASONS AND THAT HAS AFFECTED HIS COWORKERS' LIVELIHOOD!!**

The simple solution is to replace him. If I behaved like Charlie has behaved, I would, indeed, be fired, terminated, axed, canned, let go, replaced, and **FIRED** (again!). Why? Because you cannot get away with being bigger than the job. If you do not comply with what is asked of you by your employer, then you will not be employed. End of story.

CBS can and should fire Sheen. And replace him with…not a monkey. That was my way of getting the attention of the masses (and CBS). But replace him with any of the hundreds of talented, working actors out there looking for a break.

That's why I suggest that CBS have a reality-themed show designed to replace Sheen. Find ten hungry, talented, funny, out-of-work actors, put them all in one apartment, and have one replace Sheen each week on *"Two and a Half Men."* At the end of the ten-week talent search, and after creating a ratings powerhouse, the new "Charlie" is revealed. Everybody wins. The current cast of the show, who, because of the selfish antics of their star are not making a living, get to work and get paid. And someone new on the horizon, as good as but more than likely better than Sheen, gets his shot at stardom.

And best yet, the audience, you out there who need laughter to end your day after having to scrape and toil for your daily bread and gasoline, you, my friend, gets to chuckle during dinner, a necessary respite, delivered by a fresh face, hopefully sans chemicals and attitude, that will make you smile…and not give a moment's thought to Carlos Estevez.

Life is too short to put up with the Charlie Sheen's of the world. Think about it. If this guy lived next door to you or, heaven forbid, were related to you, would you allow him to continue with such bizarre, destructive, and repugnant behavior? No, you would see that he seeks help…and change the channel, in hope of discovering something to take your mind off your troubles. And have a jolly chortle or two in the meantime.

Until next time…

peace,

Mike

SAYING GOODBYE TO THE END OF A VERY BAD YEAR

I hadn't planned on writing an end of the year article in 2008, certainly not while December was still in its early stages. But, more often than not, life gets in the way of many of our best laid plans. And, sad to say, death does too.

2008 has not been a good year. For me, personally, and for most of the world, it seems that this year is one for the books in terms of bad news.

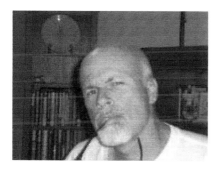

My wife and I, like millions of others (dare I say, billions?), have seen our net worth reduced by numbers too large and ugly to put into print. Yet we remain employed, still have the wherewithal to earn decent livings, and are thankful for that. But millions of others are unemployed, and from all the forecasts things will certainly get worse before they get better.

But even though those are big challenges to overcome, it's only money, right? At least you have your health…right?

2008 has been a trying year health-wise for me. My left shoulder began acting up early in the year, to the point where it needed to be surgically repaired, and still is far from one hundred percent. Yet I am thankful that the rest of me is okay. But that's just me. And it's only a sore shoulder. Things could be worse.

What if that sore shoulder turned out to be something bigger? It's not, but, again, that's just me--I got lucky. Sadly, my brother and his new bride did not.

One of my best memories of this past year was being asked to participate in my brother's wedding. In a year often filled with gloom and doom, this joyous event was a nice respite from the darkness. Yet for all its happiness, that day had a foreboding shrouding the event. My new sister-in-law, a lovely bride and the sparkle in my brother's eye, was sick. They pushed up their nuptials by several months to accommodate her illness. Life and its paradoxes. 2008, that dreadful, yet wonderful, year.

They remain deeply in love and are hanging in there, both doing all that they can to make the best of their situation, doing what we humans often do when facing adversity: persevere, deal and cope, live life.

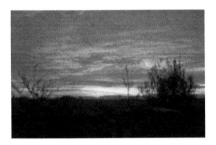

Life.

And death.

The reason I am writing this today is due to having to fly Back East in a few days to attend a funeral. My step-father, one of the kindest, nicest men I have had the pleasure to meet, and a wonderful companion for my mother over the past eleven years, succumbed to illness and age on the anniversary of the Pearl Harbor invasion. This is significant given that he fought in that war, returned with a wound and a determination to live life to its fullest every day. Which he did for eighty-eight years. My entire family are better people for having known him. And my mom? She's tough, a survivor. But recovering from losing your love, that person with whom you share your daily existence, takes time.

It will take well into next year, and possibly the next, to fully recover from the many loses felt during this trying year. And that is what this is really about, what livelife365.com is all about.

Living your life

Every day

Every way

Not letting anyone (or anything)

Stand in your way.

In memory of my step-father, in honor of my mother, with love to my brother, his wife, and the rest of my family (especially my wife and my son [Happy Birthday, Kiddo!]), and to all those who lost someone or something dear to them during this troubling year, I offer you my latest song, "livelife365":

Life struggles by

Another dream left to die

But no matter what the fates have in mind

You still try

Turn the page

Live your life every day

Don't let anybody stand in your way

Work it out

Grab the bull by the horns

Make it count

Choose the rose not the thorns

Fight for your dreams

Even when it all seems

No one believes anyway

Live your life every day

Make a choice

Use your voice

Have your say

Don't let anybody stand in your way

Life carries on

Another dream has been born

Touch the sky so glad you're alive

Livelife365

I hope this inspires you, as it does me, to live your life to its fullest every day. And while 2008 has not been one of the better years in recent memory, it has been a year in your life. Good or bad, it's your life. Your year. And it should be remembered for that.

Peace,

Mike

HOW TO SURVIVE AN ELECTION-YEAR FINANCIAL MELTDOWN

I know what some of you are saying, *"Why should I listen to what you have to say about the economy? You're a self-help guy, who specializes in healthy lifestyle and personal development, as well as makes funny (goofy) videos and goofy (funny) parody songs."*

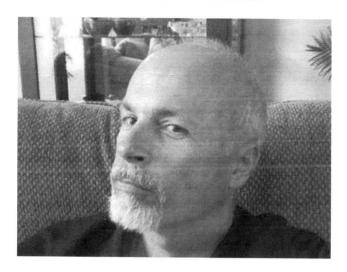

Why? Because in dire times like these (seen the Business headlines recently?), during the most important presidential election of our lifetime, it takes a commonsense and practical approach to combat all the craziness going on out there.

Q: But, Mike, you write and make videos about diet and nutrition, motivation and how-to, what do you know about finances?

A: As much as the next guy, and more than enough to help you.

TEN THINGS YOU CAN DO TO SURVIVE THE ELECTION YEAR FINANCIAL MELTDOWN

1. DON'T PANIC

Wall Street seems to feed on panic—panic buying and panic selling. While others overreact and sell off their stocks and put their cash in <u>safer investments</u>, you don't need to follow suit. Unless you need the money from those investments right now, standing pat is still the best option. Why? Because stocks eventually *ALWAYS* come back up—this is an historical fact. And if they don't, then we're all in trouble. This too shall pass.

2. SIT ON IT

Rarely, as a self-help, fitness guru, do I suggest sitting back and doing nothing. But, in this case, go right ahead! Pass the popcorn and park it on the couch. Okay, you still need your daily exercise, but with regards to your money—*LEAVE IT ALONE*. Sit on it. In fact, the best advice that I hear the most from those that get paid to know this sort of thing is: *DO NOT* stop contributing to your 401k or IRA. Why? Right now stocks are cheap. When the market goes down, prices go down. The more stock you purchase **NOW**, at lower prices, the more you will have *LATER*, when the market stabilizes and goes back up. Think about it.

3. **KISS (KEEP IT SIMPLE, SHERLOCK!)**

Simplify your life. Cut back, spend less. Analyze what you *NEED* versus what you *WANT*. If you dine out 3-4 times a week, cut that in half. Do you really need satellite TV and radio? The recent trend now is stay-at-home vacations--you spend less on gas and airfare, while discovering local attractions you may have been missing, or avoiding, for years.

Bottom line: Simplify your life and save money.

4. TAKE A WALK

How much do you spend a year on that health club membership? Figure out a way to stay in shape at home, and cancel that costly membership. <u>Walking</u> is one of the least expensive, but most effective, ways to stay in shape. Plus, it gets you outside, and is good for the mind and spirit. In times like these, that's a good thing.

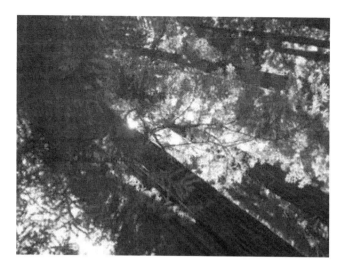

If you desire a more strenuous workout, look into purchasing dumbbells, a stationary bike or other equipment; whatever fits your specific needs. The initial investment may smart a little at first, but will more than pay for itself for years and years.

5. INVEST IN YOURSELF

While exercise and keeping fit are vital aspects of personal growth, don't stop there. Continue working on self-improvement and personal development all the time. livelife365 can help.

6. LISTEN TO YOUR BOSS

There is no place continued growth is more important right now than in the job market. Now is not the time to take your job for granted. Nor is it the time to mess up the job you have. Yes, keep that resume handy and continue networking and sharpening your skills so that you are more marketable. But you also need to keep your boss happy with your work. Work harder. Do the best job you can to make yourself indispensable. Most companies will have cutbacks and layoffs—*YOU* cannot control this. But you *CAN* control your effort, productivity, and attitude.

ALWAYS be in the *TOP* ranked twenty percent of good performers, not the bottom twenty.

Why? *GOOD* companies seldom layoff *GOOD* employees.

Be good, listen to your boss!

7. STOP AND SMELL THE FLOWERS

Enjoy yourself. Enjoy each day. Live life 365. This simply means to live your life every day in every way. Yes, times are tough, the economy is a mess, the world is a bigger mess, but you can still find a way to enjoy the little things in life that have nothing to do with the bigger things that are out of your control.

Every Day Every Way

8. GET YOUR HANDS DIRTY

Now is the time to roll up those sleeves and get to work. But you're already working on self and your job; what next? Go outside, dig up the garden. If you don't have a garden, start one. Landscape. Mow the lawn. Do house repairs, spring or fall cleaning. Learn a new (inexpensive) hobby. Do it yourself. Besides saving you a ton of money, DIY is good for the mind, body, and spirit. A sense of self-accomplishment goes a long way. And if you're picking ripe tomatoes off the vine, you're not worrying about Wall Street. Besides, growing your own will save you more money in the long run (and they taste so much better, too!). Can, bottle, preserve, or freeze whatever you can't consume now, and have a winter of homegrown, inexpensive veggies.

9. BALANCE YOURSELF

And your portfolio. The only movement you should be doing with your portfolio is rebalancing it. This simply means you need to take a look at your asset allocations. When there are sharp fluctuations in the stock market, your assets will also shift. But do me a favor, check with your financial consultant before you do anything.

As for you and *YOUR* balance: you should always be working on managing your Triad of Balance, the harmonic balance between *Mind, Body*, and *Spirit*.

10. VOTE FOR CHANGE

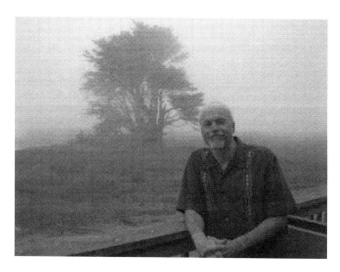

Now, more than ever, we need some major changes in Washington. If *YOU* do not like what is happening in *YOUR* life due to decisions made by our political leaders, *YOU* have the power to *CHANGE* it.

The current financial meltdown we are witnessing needs to be fixed. Fixed fast! We have the choice to keep on making the same mistakes that have led us here.

Or opt for *CHANGE*.

For the better.

I hope these tips help make dealing with these turbulent times a bit easier. And always remember that *YOU* have more power than you think to *CHANGE* your *LIFE*.

peace,

Mike

A MERE INCONVENIENCE

I sit in semi-darkness, the haunting wail of the relentless wind serenading me, periodically interrupted by the steady rat-a-tat-tat of raindrops pouring down from the heavens and belting my skylight.

The lights had been flickering, winking on and off, and then vanished completely, taken away on the angry wind, along with the rest of my electrical power, dissipating like the last hapless breaths of a terminal patient.

The house is without power, eerily quiet sans the constant thrum of the 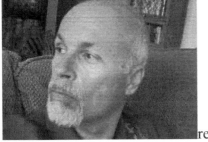refrigerator, the whir of a fan, the comforting purr of the heater rumbling into life. A severe winter storm, packed with copious amounts of cold rain and wind gusts approaching seventy miles per hour, has left my little corner of the world trapped inside its own little emergency. A mere inconvenience, really, when compared with what is happening in other areas of the world:

- War in Afghanistan
- Terrorism and unrest in Iraq
- Poverty, starvation and genocide in many African Nations
- And, most recently, the massive earthquake that devastated Haiti

Most of us are very lucky; we will survive the odd blackout with maybe only a handful of angst: some spoiled food from a warming fridge; a sniffle or two from sleeping without heat; a missed day's wage; a few hours without television or video games.

But to call losing your power for a few hours, or days, an emergency, a catastrophe, or anything more than a mere inconvenience, when placed next to the hardship those sad souls in Haiti went through, are going through, and will continue to go through is, is tantamount to comparing a mosquito bite to open heart surgery; there is no comparison.

By candlelight, I write this, with the hope that eventually the power will be restored and I can transfer my handwritten words onto my computer, and then post them to my blog. Yes, the power will eventually return, as will normal life as we know it. But what about those Haitians? Or those countless suffering human beings who live in those other war torn and impoverished nations? When will their lives return to "normal"? And, more to the point, what can we do to help them?

Give. Of yourself. Of your heart. Of your soul. And, especially, of your wallet. One dollar or one thousand, give whatever you can afford…and then give a little bit more. Give to the people of the island nation of Haiti, yes, but give to any human being who will go hungry one day (including many right here in America) or who is suffering.

And when you've given as much money as you can, then give something else: give your positive energy, your prayers, your goodwill, your love, and if you are able to, your time. I am a firm believer that giving from your heart and soul is as valuable as giving from your wallet. But give both.

This writing was inspired by a tragic front page event, but the need to help others less fortunate than most of us is always there.

One of the things that constantly amazes me about people is how, more often than not, they rise above expectations, especially in the worst of times. It happened when the towers went down on that horrible September day in 2001, and it is happening now in the aftermath of that 7.0 earthquake in Haiti. People rise to the occasion, go above and beyond, often enduring difficult sacrifices, to help those who cannot help themselves. But these amazing acts of decency are topped by the countless acts of courage and patience and perseverance exhibited by those struck by the very same tragic events others go out of their way to help combat.

Remember: Give, of your heart, your soul, and your wallet. And then give some more.

peace,

Mike

WHY SO ANGRY?

I have been writing about a lot of deep issues lately—spirituality, life, death, introspection, the tragic devastation in Haiti—and vowed that the next post I write would be one of my funny ones (hey, at least I find

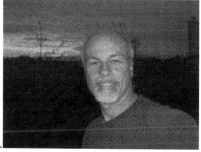

them funny). Or maybe a musical interlude that helps take your mind off all of those heavy issues crowding one another on the front pages of the newspapers, Internet, and television news.

I mean, one of the things I have always stressed at livelife365.com is the need to laugh, to enjoy life while working hard and doing all that you can to keep that old triad balanced. Life is often a struggle, filled with heartbreak and sadness. But it is also, more often than not, a beautiful, magical, wonderful experience. Oh, the paradoxes!

But while my funny post never materialized, this did:

WHY SO ANGRY?

I know things seem bad these days, in many ways for many people. To that I say: get in line! Join the club! Deal with it!

Again: **WHY SO ANGRY?**

Life is life is life. It's going to have its ups and downs, its highs and lows, its good and bad. None of this is any news, or should come as a big surprise. And I understand that lots of what's going on in the world is frustrating and totally out of your control, leading me, again, to ask:

WHY SO ANGRY?

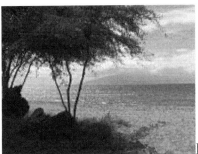Because, the way I look at it, if you react with **ANGER** to bad situations, to all those lists of things that bug you, you're going to be **ANGRY** pretty much all the time. Why would you choose to live your life that way?

I keep hearing the talking heads on the tube refer to people and their **ANGER**, how everyone is **ANGRY** with that politician so they voted him out; or how this poor guy lost his job and is now very **ANGRY**; or how this group didn't get what they wanted and they are described as, you guessed it, ANGRY.

WHY SO ANGRY?

I'm not trying to be argumentative (and, of course, this is making you **ANGRIER**, right?), I'm just saying: you choose to be **ANGRY**. The issues in this world that are making you upset and mad and **ANGRY** will be around long after we are all deep in the ground…life, as I say, is life is life. To get **ANGRY** at it, no matter how upsetting it can make us, is not the solution.

Take a look at how the dictionary defines **ANGER**:

1. strong feeling of displeasure and belligerence aroused by a wrong; wrath; ire.

And some synonyms: resentment, exasperation; choler, bile, spleen. **FURY, INDIGNATION, RAGE** imply deep and strong feelings aroused by injury, injustice, wrong, etc.

Wow, pretty intense, huh? Leading me to interject once again:

WHY SO ANGRY?

Here's how I look at it—I get it, I see the big picture. There is frustration out there: healthcare reform, unemployment, racism, terrorism, bungling politicians, overpaid executives, greedy bankers—I'm not blind or unsympathetic to those issues. But to react to them with **ANGER**, hatred or anything but trying to seek positive solutions makes you, well, part of the problem.

It's easy to point fingers, say "I told you so," and embrace the negative movement propagated by too many for reasons that are beyond me. To basically sit and get **ANGRY** versus taking action and trying to change things...well, to that I say:

WHY NOT DO SOMETHING ABOUT IT?

Getting angry serves no purpose. In fact, it can cause serious health problems—heart attacks, high blood pressure, depression, violence. Getting angry is how narrow minded, uncreative, do-nothings react to problems. We all have problems. We all have days, weeks, sometimes years, when things go wrong and our lives seem hopeless. We deserve to be down, right?

"We are judged by how we react to adversity more than how we embrace prosperity."

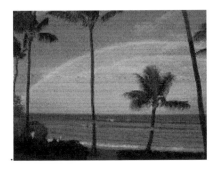

It's good to have passion, to care, to be informed; don't ever stop living your life with purpose. But **ANGER**? No.

Take all that **ANGER**, please, and try to channel it, put it to constructive, positive use, and, guess what? You may just discover that you will gradually become part of the solution and not the problem. And, better yet:

YOU MAY NO LONGER BE ANGRY.

Think about it.

Smile.

peace,

Mike

MODULATE, PLEASE!

Who are these people? You know the ones, those loud-talkers that call attention to themselves in places that were once civil and respectable establishments.

Take this recent dining experience—I'm sitting with the one I love, sifting through my salad, enjoying *"normal"* conversation, when this sudden noise, this garish shriek of uninteresting garbage, this overloud television commercial of a human being intrudes upon my space to share their day's events with me, instead of quietly with the person across from them.

I find myself asking an unanswerable question: ***"Why does this clueless fool feel the need to share their banal personal life with the rest of us?"***

Sadly, I always conclude with the obvious:

"Because they appear to indeed be clueless."

At least I hope that's why. Because if ignorance is not the reason for being one of those loud-talking louts who interrupt (dare I say sabotage?) decent social behavior, then the only other conclusion would be selfishness, rudeness, or maybe just plain mean arrogance.

That is a rather frightening thought.

To those scary souls I say:

"MODULATE, PLEASE!"

But it's not just in restaurants, not just clueless loud-talkers, sharing endless streams of trite drivel. How about those cell phone gum-flappers? Or those parents who publicly scream at their kids? You know the ones that must be suffering from a mild case of amnesia, thinking that they are in their living rooms as they demand that little Sally or Bobby—for the tenth time!—pick

up that toy **RIGHT NOW! ONE…TWO**…Don't make me count to
THREE!

There is a rudeness going around these days, like a virus, only one with no
hypodermic needle available as a remedy for this bizarre epidemic. I say
bizarre because the solution is simple manners, common decency, and the
ability to differentiate between acceptable public behavior and the
unacceptable.

But that's just it. Sadly, again, I am not sure enough people actually
understand what acceptable public behavior is anymore.

"MODULATE, PLEASE!"

Blame can be doled out in several places, starting with the breakdown of
family values. These things need to be taught at home, at the beginning of
one's early development, as necessary as learning to read or walk.

Technology is an easy target. After all, with electronic communication and
social networking readily available at the touch of one's fingertips, folks
feel that the world is in their living rooms. But is that any excuse for
selfish, rude, intrusive behavior? Sadly, again, it is not.

Frankly, I'm befuddled. Because while I embrace having the world at my
doorstep and fingertips, I have never used my cell phone in an intrusive,
rude, or selfish manner. Never imagined doing so.

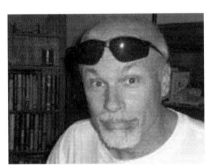

Leading me to conclude that this problem—be it loud-talkers in public
places, rude cell phone barkers, heavy bass music blarers, or oversaturated
cologne and perfume spritzers—is linked to the spirit, the essence of our
existence. Basic tenets of decency taught to most of us…but somehow
recently forgotten.

Simple, basic—**HUMAN**—behavioral traits like:

· Kindness
· Unselfishness
· Being charitable
· Politeness
· Giving
· Sharing
· Considerate
· Common decency

Anyone who argues that they are all of the above yet exhibit any of the sad behavior mentioned in this post are not only fooling themselves, but polluting the world.

Think about it.

peace (and quiet),

Mike

ENTERTAINMENT

III. ETC.

THROUGH DEATH WE LEARN ABOUT LIFE

This past Saturday marked nineteen years since my father passed away.

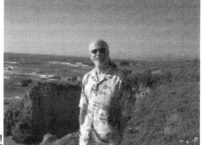

Nineteen years! I will never forget the haunting wail of that early morning telephone call from my brother, the ominous sensation tugging at my flesh as my fingers found the receiver and I knew that nothing good would come from my lifting it to my groggy head. My goodness, I had brown hair back then, and it filled the majority of my skull! I was living in Southern California, in the midst of another bad marriage, juggling several vices that were on the threshold of dragging me down into a hole of depression and angst that would take me years to climb out of.

Nineteen years.

While the pain is no longer fresh, the grief not as insurmountable as it once seemed, the loss, the void my father's passing left in me, is as substantial now as it was then. Sure, I can conjure up a good sob every once and a while, whenever the mood beckons and I feel the need to let go. But while way back in the day those bouts of sadness were often accompanied by fits of anger at my father for not taking better care of himself, and then guilt, for not cutting my old man a break, I have grown from the experience, changed for the better.

Nineteen years.

You see, my father's death, while still one of the most awful events that has

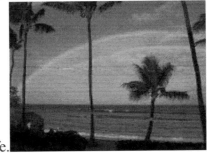

ever affected me, changed my life. His
death, in fact, could be said to have created livelife365. And while I would
give anything to have him back in my life again, enjoying his
companionship and influence, watching him age as gracefully as my
mother, I do not dwell on his death; not anymore. As I said, my father's
death changed my life.

My father was very human, meaning he had many flaws, like we all do.
He was a heavy drinker, a lifelong smoker, someone who overindulged
in more than a few meals, and often struggled to make ends meet. He
died well before his time, in my mind at least, just midway into his
fifties (only a few years older than I am). But he also instilled in me the
self-confidence and belief in myself that has helped to make me the man
I am today. As a young boy I can still feel the power of my father's
motivational words, telling me that I could be anything I wanted to
be…as long as I believed in myself.

But it was my father's vices, more that his attributes, that prompted me
to change my life for the better. Not long after he died, I took inventory
of myself and did not like what I saw. I was overweight, boozing it up,
smoking, depressed, in a bad marriage (another one), working at a job
that I did not like, and, literally, wasting my time on earth. His death, at
first, only made me worse—I actually started drinking more, if that was
possible (yes, it was, by the way), and fell into a deeper depression.

And then something snapped inside me. It was the first Father's Day
after he died. I had hit all-time lows with my drinking, smoking,
overeating, job performance; I was separated from my wife and son,
living in a one-room apartment, seeing a therapist that wasn't helping.

Somehow I found an inner strength that had always been there, just buried through years and years of confusion and abuse.

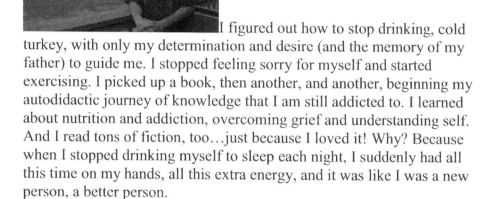 I figured out how to stop drinking, cold turkey, with only my determination and desire (and the memory of my father) to guide me. I stopped feeling sorry for myself and started exercising. I picked up a book, then another, and another, beginning my autodidactic journey of knowledge that I am still addicted to. I learned about nutrition and addiction, overcoming grief and understanding self. And I read tons of fiction, too…just because I loved it! Why? Because when I stopped drinking myself to sleep each night, I suddenly had all this time on my hands, all this extra energy, and it was like I was a new person, a better person.

I changed my life through my dad's death.

Nineteen years.

There have been plenty of ups and downs throughout those nineteen years, several other lifestyle changes and challenges. But some things have never changed, and those are my thoughts on the importance of life. Not wasting your life. Not allowing anything to get in the way of doing all that you want and have to do with the precious time we have on earth

But also understanding that life is life. It can be as cruel and uncertain as it is wondrous and rewarding. It is up to each of us to take what we can from it, while never taking it for granted or expecting from it anything that is not earned through sweat and tears and compassion and love.

My dad died nineteen years ago this past week and it was the worst thing that ever happened to me. And the best. The lessons he taught me while alive, while valuable and influential, were nothing compared to what he taught me through his death.

Rest in peace, Dad. I love you.

peace,

Mike

VOLUNTEERING ON VACATION

Whenever I go on vacation, I have simple objectives, most of them related to how much rest and relaxation I can cram into my days away

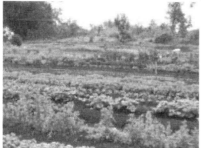

from it all. Oh, sure, I also love discovering new places and different things to do, wining and dining, spending quality time with my lovely wife, and catching up on my reading.

But I am also at the stage in my life where I crave doing more, even while lolling in the sun, listening to the crash of endless waves and gazing off into the nothingness without a care in the world. Yes, even while on a tropical paradise like Maui, I try to manage my triad of

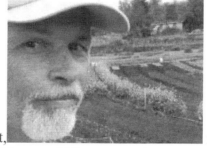

balance—I exercise, eat right, read and write every day, and look inside myself for personal growth opportunities that enhance my spirituality.

This year, while perusing one of those guides you pick up at the airport that brag about dozens of great things to do while in Hawaii, I stumbled upon one of the most rewarding experiences my wife and I have shared and enjoyed in ages.

I phoned the Pacific Whale Foundation and learned that not only could they offer us such amazing adventures like a day of working at an organic farm in the upcountry town of Kula, or helping remove invasive species at sacred, protected grounds in the West Maui Mountains,

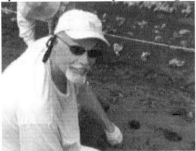 but that they wouldn't cost a cent, not one Maui dollar. Not only that, by volunteering to get our hands dirty and our bodies sweaty, we could also meet wonderful people, experience new and interesting activities, and feel that incredible feeling that only giving of your time for a worthy cause can give you.

I have to say that I have been fortunate enough to have visited Maui many times, and while every visit is special and enjoyable, this visit, and our volunteering efforts, was the highlight of decades of highlights. We gave back, added solutions to problems by participating in organic farming, socialized with like-minded, friendly people, and even finagled a free farm-fresh lunch out of the deal.

Here is a brief snapshot of my day at O'o farm:

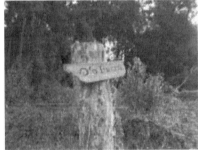

- · awoke at 6:00 am
- · drove to upcountry town of Pukalani
- · met with other volunteers
- · met Richard and Sunanda at O'o Farm
- · assigned to pull weeds for a few hours with Sunanda

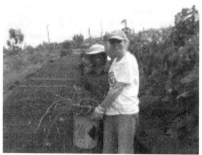

- watched others pull weeds while I filmed
- watched others pull weeds while I made Sunanda laugh
- filled wheelbarrow with weeds
- emptied wheelbarrow filled with weeds
- stopped for lunch
- made Sunanda laugh
- enjoyed an amazing homemade vegetarian meal made by Sunanda
- happily discovered a port-o-potty
- went back to work at the farm
- watched Wendy and Brenda and Sunanda plant vegetables
- filmed them planting vegetables
- firmly told to put the camera away and help plant vegetables
- happily discovered the port-o-potty again
- stopped and gazed at the amazing vista of the Pacific ocean from several thousand feet above sea level
- announced to all, for the hundredth time, how content, pleased, thrilled, fulfilled, and excited I was to be sharing such a

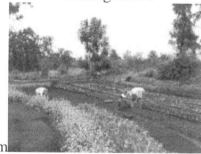

  wonderful experience with them
- planted some vegetables
- shot some video
- made Sunanda laugh again
- and called it a day

Volunteering any time is an important way to give back to those who are less fortunate than us, as well as helping others who are working to change the world for the better. Volunteering while on vacation makes something that is great to begin with even more so. And adds a spiritual balance to the rest of your life.

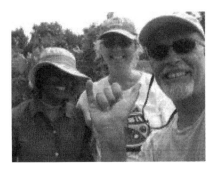

I would like to thank everyone at the Pacific Whale Foundation and O'o Farm, Brenda, and especially Richard, Sunanda, and Dasa, who went out of their way to make my wife and I feel as if we'd known them forever, and whom we now consider forever friends.

peace,

Mike

LANDSCAPE ESCAPE

I'm one of those lucky guys who have lots of hobbies to occupy my time

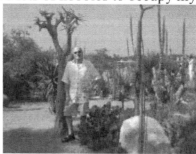

and energy. I am an avid reader and
collector of books (as well as tea and turtles). I love to travel and play
my guitar. And I stay busy with my writing, videos, and music projects.
But one of my favorite hobbies is landscaping. I like nothing better than
to take an empty or weed-strewn chunk of land and turn it into a
colorful, blooming masterpiece that enhances the natural scenery and
makes me smile every time I wander through it.

I enjoy landscaping so much that I consider it therapeutic, one of my
great escapes whenever I need some time away from the everyday
challenges and all too often stresses of life.

Besides being a terrific form of exercise, landscaping is a wonderful
way to get back to nature, to roll up those sleeves and dig your hands
into the earth. There's nothing like working up a sweat with the sounds
of birds or squirrels singing and chirping away in the background.

Another thing that draws me to landscaping is the sense of
accomplishment I feel when I (finally) complete a project. Life is a
journey that should be enjoyed throughout each leg; the same can be
said about landscaping. I like the fact that there's a beginning, middle,
and end, and while the finish line can seem a long way off at the outset
of any project, the key is to enjoy every minute of the experience--I do
this with landscaping, just as I try to do with all aspects of my life.

One thing I always talk about trying to achieve is the *Triad of Balance*,
which is working on finding harmony between the *Mind*, *Body*, and
Spirit, after first balancing each one on its own. Simply put: in order to
lead the most fulfilling and purposeful life, I believe one has to work on

the **Mind**, **Body**, and **Spirit** every day, and then balance all three

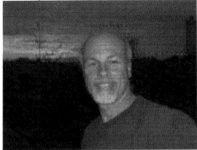

together. If one of these is out of whack, then even though the other two are working fine, you are not complete, not in balance, and, therefore, not living your life to its fullest. Landscaping is one of those hobbies that helps me to stay balanced. My **MIND** is in constant motion, thinking and planning, focused on the tasks at hand and then executing and achieving. While my **SPIRIT** feels free as I dig up the dirt, plant flowers and trees, communing with nature. I also feel less stressful: when I am outside with a shovel in my hands I seldom allow distractions to interfere--a good thing. Lastly, my **BODY** gets plenty of work pushing a wheelbarrow around, freeing up boulders from the ground, and digging, digging, digging. Landscaping is great exercise and a calorie burner.

So what are you waiting for? Summer may be over, but fall is an excellent time to do some planting and work around the yard. Besides being a fun and rewarding hobby, landscaping is a chance to help you find balance between your **MIND**, **BODY**, and **SPIRIT**. Think about it.

peace,

Mike

LIVING ABOVE YOUR MEANS

Stuff. Things. Possessions.

We all like to buy stuff, right? As a self-admitted <u>collector</u>, there's
nothing I enjoy more than perusing a quaint used bookstore in search of
a rare first edition to complete a collected set of one of my favorite
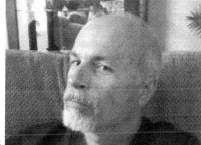
authors.

We work hard all day, why not splurge a little and go for that extra-
extra, big-big flat screen HDTV, right? Or take that expensive vacation
to the Mediterranean. Or opt for an extra 500 square feet and the three-
car garage for that stunning house in that gated community.

Why not?

You deserve it.

Or do you?

Merit. Deserve. Entitlement.

I want it all! Now!

Living **ABOVE** your means.

The recent credit crunch, housing market bubble burst, and subsequent
Wall Street meltdown has made all of us more cognizant of our
financial situations. But all these financial fireworks and government
bailouts and foreclosures and job losses and political promises and

401K angst have one major connection, one common thread:

PEOPLE LIVING ABOVE THEIR MEANS!

I like to compare those living above their means to someone who is grossly overweight, knows they need to change, but just keeps eating too much of the wrong foods until they eventually face dire health (and all too often catastrophic financial) consequences.

They need help.

They need to learn to "budget" their caloric intake. Need to understand why they *THINK* they *NEED* to eat the wrong foods and the wrong amounts. Same thing goes for those overspending, being financially careless.

They need to <u>live within their means.</u>

While practicing better fitness and nutrition is always a major focus of mine at <u>livelife365.com</u>, this particular chapter deals more with financial responsibility and personal accountability.

Just as the politicians, during the recently completed (it IS over, right?) presidential campaign, pounded the need for change into our heads, we, too, need to make changes in the way WE do things. But, guess what?

Change is good!

Is change easy?

That's another story. Change can be painful, difficult, challenging, but no less painful or challenging as filing for bankruptcy. Or having your house foreclosed on. Or having to ignore a medical condition because you can't afford to visit a doctor.

Here are some ways to help you try to live within your means:

- **ADMIT** you have a problem. Take personal accountability and understand that you **CAN'T AFFORD** everything that you **WANT**. Hey, I would love another 500 square feet and a nifty three-car garage, but will not put myself into unnecessary debt just to have it.
- **BUDGET YOURSELF**. Go on a financial diet. Just like when dieting to lose unwanted pounds, this is easier said than done. What can you do?
- **EDUCATE YOURSELF**. Visiting websites like livelife365.com, is a great start, but don't stop there. Read, read, and read some more. Ask questions to qualified financial experts every chance you get. The more you know the better ability you have to understand your particular financial situation, what you can and cannot afford. You should know how much of a mortgage you can afford BEFORE you ever sit down across from a member of any lending institution. If you don't, then you're probably not ready to buy a house.
- **THINK LAYAWAY**. Before the human race became consumed with credit, they used to pay for things **BEFORE** they bought them. This not only gives you a wonderful sense of accomplishment and appreciation, but it also keeps you out of unwanted and sometimes devastating debt. It helps you…

LIVE WITHIN YOUR MEANS.

In a way, living a layaway life is the antithesis of being under the misguided misconception of feeling compelled to have a life of entitlement.

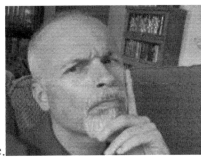

Simply put: We need to change.

Change the way we think.

Change the way we spend.

Yes, change the way we eat (had to throw that one in).

Change the way we live.

There's a lot of nice stuff out there, things and possessions that we all think we need and can't live without. But unless you really, really need something or at least can easily afford it, then the solution is simple:

Just say no.

And try to change your life…for the better.

peace,

Mike

I FEEL YOUR PAIN

I am normally an active person. I was one of those kids who couldn't sit still, was always on the go and in constant motion. Probably drove my parents crazy. This frenetic energy followed me into adulthood.

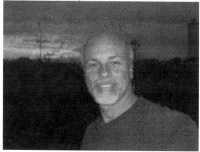

I like to keep moving and, given that for most of my working life I find myself situated in front of this computer for hours on end, I make sure I find the time to exercise daily: walking, bike riding, lifting weights, calisthenics, or just working around the house.

Staying active has suited me well these many decades. Nothing like the comfortable ache of pushing and testing your muscles and joints with good, hard effort, then rewarding yourself with a soothing hot shower, an enjoyable meal, and relaxation with family and friends at the end of the day. But a lot of that has changed for me recently.

What if those comfortable aches begin to linger? Or if those sore muscles and joints remain sore long after what is considered a "normal" period of recovery?

I feel your pain.

In fact, I feel _my pain_. For months now, I have been battling chronic shoulder pain. It hurts to do just about anything that involves using my left shoulder.

The sad fact is, my shoulder is filled with pain, especially when I use it a certain way. And since the pain radiates along my entire arm, it even hurts when I write.

Being a man, and by that I mean being a stubborn creature who only visits a doctor as a last resort, I first ignored the pain, hoping that it would go away, like most aches and sore muscles eventually do. When it did not, I added aspirin and a heating pad to my home remedy. Still no improvement, so I added constant complaining and moaning to my inept self-healing cure. Again, no change. So I had this conversation with my wife:

Mike: My shoulder is killing me!

Wife: Go see a doctor.

Mike: I don't know what to do anymore.

Wife: Go see a doctor.

Mike: I mean, I've tried everything…

Wife: Go see a doctor.

Mike: It's never felt like this before.

Wife: Go see a doctor.

Mike: It really hurts.

Wife: Go see a doctor.

Mike: Think I should go see a doctor?

Wife glares at Mike, sadly shaking her head as she walks out of the room.

I finally take my lovely wife's advice and visit my doctor. This begins a chain of events that takes me from x-rays to physical therapy to a botched MRI to more PT to a cortisone injection to another MRI to weeping like a small child to more physical therapy to one more cortisone injection to sucking my thumb in the fetal position to one last trip to my physical therapist (who my wife now thinks I am secretly dating) to…today.

Or should I say: tomorrow.

Thursday, October 16, 2008, I will be having arthroscopic surgery to repair the pain in my left shoulder.

I look forward to this procedure with paradoxical caution: I am not thrilled with the prospect of being anesthetized and having someone poke around my bursa, bones, muscle, and what-have-you, but on the other hand I am tired of the pain and ready to remedy it.

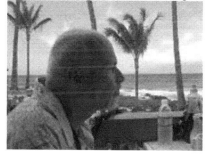

I leave you with this thought to ponder while I am recovering:

Listen to your body. That comfortable ache after exercise or physical activity is a good thing, an indication that you have been active and your muscles and joints are happy and healing. But if that ache lingers or turns into something more, then do yourself a favor and listen to your wife.

Go see a doctor.

peace,

Mike

BEAT THOSE WINTER BLUES

Where's the sun? Is it freezing in here, or is it just me? Pass the Kleenex…ah, could you hurry…ah…ahh…ahhh. Sniffle, sniffle.

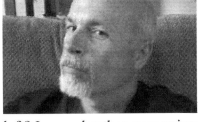Hey, are there any more holiday cookies left? Is your brother *ever* going to leave our guest bedroom? Man, I feel like…hold on…ah…ahhh…ahhhh

CHOOOO!

Winter. Blah.

Is it spring yet?

Nope, not for a long time.

Does this sound familiar? This time of year, after weeks of overindulging on fattening foods during the holidays, compounded by icy and sun-deprived weather, further complicated by the cold and flu season, can take its toll. Hey, I can go on and on, complain with the best of them. Instead, I'd rather offer up some positive tips on how to:

<u>BEAT THOSE WINTER BLUES</u>

TAKE A HIKE!

Or at least take a walk. Too cold or rainy outside? That does present some problems, but ones that need to be addressed if you not only want to help combat those winter blues, but stay (get?) in shape. A daily thirty-minute walk does wonders for you. It gets your blood flowing, which actually warms you up, shaking the cobwebs off the old bones and sending much needed (and appreciated) endorphins to the brain that stimulate your soul (and life) with happiness. Still too cold for you? Get yourself a treadmill or stationary bike, anything! Just pump those legs and pump that blood. Be sure to dress accordingly: hat, gloves, waterproof jacket, and, always, good walking shoes.

STEP AWAY FROM THE COOKIES!

Eating the right foods and the right amounts is a reoccurring mantra for me. There is no better time to adopt healthier nutritional eating habits than right now, during the blah winter months, following the holiday (overindulging) season. Besides assisting your weight loss goals (and we all have those, don't we?), proper nutrition can actually make you FEEL better

PASS THE KLEENEX AND WASH YOUR HANDS!

Sneezing, coughing, phlegm-laden human beings that you come into contact with are everywhere this time of year, and often unavoidable. But you **CAN** protect yourself from catching whatever illness is ailing them by following a few precautions:

- Try to avoid shaking hands or having other contact if you know someone is sick.
- Wash your hands with HOT water and soap throughout the day. If you can't, then carry a hand sanitizer with you and use that until you can wash properly.
- Cover your mouth and nose when you sneeze, hoping that others will do the same for you.
- Always use a Kleenex, and toss it when done. Don't use hankies, they hold germs.
- Wash your hands **BEFORE** and **AFTER** using a public restroom, then use a paper towel to turn off the faucet and one for the door handle.

- Try to avoid sharing telephones, keyboards, pens--anything where hand-to-hand contact is prevalent.
- **ALWAYS** disinfect hotel room TV remote controls!

SUPPLEMENT THE SUN!

Winter weather can swallow up the sun for days on end, and that's not a good thing. Why? Vitamin D. A lack of this important vitamin, which we get naturally from exposure to the sun, can lead to myriad health issues, as well as contribute to the winter blues.

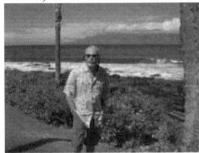 A simple solution: Take a vitamin D supplement. A not so simple solution: Move to Maui.

GRAB A GUITAR!

Sometimes boredom or the same old, same old contributes to the blahs this time of year. Why not start that hobby you've been putting off? I love playing my guitar. It helps take my mind off things and it is said that music, be it performing or just listening to it, can cheer you up. Not musically inclined? There are hundreds of other hobbies that may interest you: sewing, reading, collecting, the list is endless, the rewards many.

SMALLER IS BIGGER!

Enjoy the simpler things in life, especially during these challenging financial times. Play with your kids. Take a nice stroll with your spouse…to the bedroom. Cook a meal together. Work a puzzle, jigsaw or crossword. Interact, in positive ways, with those who mean the most to you and those winter blues will evaporate like a snowman in July (except in Canada and parts of Minnesota). Deal, adjust, cope, enjoy.

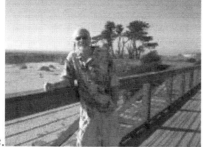

Live life.

LAUGH IT OFF!

Nothing beats humor and laughter to make those winter blah/blues go away. Laughter not only cheers you up and makes you feel better, but it's proven to be healthy for you. The significance of laughter is often underrated as a healthy option for what's bringing you down or making you sick.

Winter has just begun and will not be over any time soon. Why not make the best of winter (can you tell it's not my favorite season?) by taking action and doing everything you can to enhance each day, living life to its fullest. Every day. Every way. And beat those winter blues.

peace,

Mike

KEYS TO A HAPPY, HEALTHY GETAWAY

My wife and I just returned from a 4th of July getaway across the Sierra Nevada Mountains, to Reno. Why Reno? Well, it's close (three hours), and the drive is relaxing and filled with enjoyable scenery—mountaintops still speckled with snow, rivers cutting rapids through rock-strewn ravines, waterfalls and forests, historical bridges and quaint towns. We also like to lose ourselves with the lure of gambling, fine dining, diverse shopping, and the occasional show. It's always an easy option whenever we feel the need to escape from the everyday.

But if you are like me and have certain special dietary needs, you need to plan ahead. Here are a few tips that will help make your next getaway smoother and more rewarding:

BRING YOUR OWN

I seldom leave on a trip—short jaunt or long trek—without my trusty Bodum travel tea kettle. It's compact and light enough to fit in any carryon bag or suitcase. I suggest you also pack your tea (or coffee) cup and spoon—that way you don't have to worry about finding one in the morning, and this also reduces exposure to germs (never use those glasses they put in hotel bathrooms!). I also bring along all of my favorite green teas (as well as rooibos and yerba matte) in a Ziploc bag. If traveling by automobile, I toss in a case of mountain spring water—you can stuff six bottles at a time into your carryon or on your person and bring them up to your room. This allows you to have safe water (not all bottled waters are created equal) to drink and make tea with, as well as saving you a bunch of money. I never drink tap water, even at home—I always bring along my own spring water while dining out. And I bring it along, whenever possible, while on vacation. I enjoy Crystal Geyser or Arrowhead. It makes a difference which type you drink. Always opt for mountain spring versus purified.

For longer trips, or if traveling by air, I will pack the Bodum travel tea kettle and my own tea, but then buy a case of mountain spring water at either a grocery store or Wal-Mart, if one is convenient. The difference in cost per bottle when you buy it by the case (around 21 cents per bottle) versus purchasing a bottle in the lobby of that fancy hotel (anywhere from $2.00-$4.00 per bottle) is staggering. Spend your hard-earned cash on some fun, not bottled water. Plus, there's no guarantee that the lobby gift shop carries mountain spring water—most of the time you're paying for bottled tap water that has just been purified.

DON'T ASSUME

If you have special dietary needs (and being a pretty strict vegetarian, I sure do!), then never assume that the restaurants at the resort or city or area you are visiting will offer the same dining fare you are accustom to. The good news: most restaurants these days do offer a few vegetarian menu items to choose from—but often they lack adequate protein or fiber, or are just salads or vegetable plates.

The solution: Bring your own, if you can. I never leave on a road trip or getaway without a Trader Joe's bag filled with healthy snacks that satisfy my vegetarian needs (okay, and some fun stuff that just taste good—hey, you're on vacation, after all, right?).

But the best solution:

DO YOUR HOMEWORK

Before leaving on any trip, go online and research the area you are visiting. Search for the restaurants or hotels that cater to your special needs (and not just vegetarian needs, but whatever your particular needs may be). Unless you're vacationing in some obscure, faraway, remote island in the middle of nowhere, you should be able to find something that satisfies you.

Using the Internet (or magazines, newspaper articles, bolgs) for research before your trip is also invaluable for planning where to stay, what to do, how to get there, how much you should spend, and the best time to go.

HAVE FUN

Remember, you're getting away from your routine, the everyday. If for some reason you can't find exactly what you need to eat (I still have this challenge, at times, no matter how much planning I do), then just go with it. By that I don't mean you should scarf down a cheeseburger if you're a vegetarian. But if a burger joint is your only option, then ask if they can make you a <u>veggie burger</u>. If those aren't on the menu, try asking them for something creative, like: a cheeseburger without the burger. Maybe a side salad instead of fries (oh, what the heck, have a few fries, Mike—you're on vacation!). Or, do what I do when there is absolutely nothing that I can eat—order a salad, and then save room for dessert. I seldom eat dessert, but when I do I dive into it—banana split or slab of carrot cake. It is a getaway, after all, right?

I hope these tips help make your next getaway a happy and healthier one.

Oh, and one last thing. When gambling in Reno (or anywhere else), always set a high and a low. It's simple: if you win a jackpot, don't give it all back to the house (because the odds strongly favor this happening) by continuing to play. Set a high, and a low, dollar amount. When you hit either amount, cash in your winnings and live to gamble another day. Don't let the house win when you have the opportunity to quit while you're ahead.

On that note, think I will take my own advice.

peace,

Mike

VII. FEEDBACK

Feedback

If you have arrived at this page, I can assume that you have read my entire book—or at least skimmed through the best parts and ended up here. Or maybe you're one of those book-readers who automatically flip to the last chapter to see how it all turns out? However you got here, I still want to express my thanks and appreciation at having even purchased this book and some way or another ended up on this feedback chapter, indeed the last chapter of this book, but far from the end of the journey of self-help discovery needed to improve one's life.

My goal has always been to help as many people change their lives for the better as I can humanly reach. This book is one of the many ways I have put my message out there for hundreds of thousands (and eventually **MILLIONS**) of people. If I succeeded, something you have read over the course of these several hundred pages has grabbed you and helped you in some small (hopefully **BIG**) way. The good news, and one of the things that keeps me going, is the overwhelming outpouring of support and positive feedback I've received since I started livelife365—that means that livelife365 is working!

Over the next few pages, please enjoy some of the feedback I have received from people, just like you, who were searching for something to change their lives and found it either at my video website or blog. Who knows? Maybe your amazing story will be shared with millions in my next book.

Until next time…

peace,

Mike

HEALTH NUT WANNABEE MOM said...

> This is one of the best posts I have read anywhere. I am a vegetarian and enjoy the foods you mentioned as well. I did find the whole grain information especially helpful as I was not aware of how much protein was in that. I love soybeans and probably have them 5-6 times a week!!!

Spin Diva said...

> Awesome, awesome article!! It is so important to know the caloric content of the food we eat--it really helps in making better choices in what we eat. Thanks for sharing.

Laura-Junkfoodaholic said...

> I loved reading your article. It's very informative and easy to understand. Congratulations on losing 40 pounds and more importantly, keeping it off for two years. That's awesome!

Awesome video(s) Mike. I started looking for help for my girlfriend who's fighting cancer, and at the same time, I WANT to lose at 'least' 40 lbs. I have found your videos truly helpful and encouraging. And I'm switching my snack foods from Cheesies'n Chips, to ALMONDS :)

Thanks for making this info available Mike.

smitty747

Sir, you are an inspiration, thank you for your advice. At first i thought i could never lose ten pounds but now it seems so easy thank you so much this made me want to try harder

MusiqGirl4Ever16

Thanks for the advice i actually took the time to write the important things down. I can't wait to start this. Thanks Man You're a Life Saver

IchihaMind

Thank you so much for this video. I'm a 20 yr. old college student and I'm trying my best to change my eating habits for the better. Green tea has become my new obsession! It's begun to help me concentrate in school, helps me exercise and keeps me awake during the day. It's so nice to have that healthy pick-me-up instead of settling for those energy drinks that make me crash. You're awesome! <3

ShadowedVeil7

Howdy Mike!!

I'm really enjoying the videos you have on your channel. I love all things music and herbs!!

But in response to your video where you speak of your fathers passing, it really made me look back on my own personal experience of loss when my father died. I had a brief few moments of sadness and out of nowhere I just broke down and sobbed for a few good minutes. It wasn't as if I were back at that time in my life, but I guess it was maybe "unfinished business" so to speak, as though there were still pockets of unaddressed pain that I've somehow stomped down and buried.

Anyway, it felt good to have that unexpected emotional release. I sometimes find myself leaning more towards the "bottle it up" kind of reaction to difficult emotions (ones where tears may become involved) but I'm working on doing something about that!!

I really thought that the sunset in that video WAS very nice, such a beautiful scene. It reminded me of some of the beautifully scenic photos I used in the attached video. I thought maybe you could enjoy these awesome pictures as well. Sadly, they are only ones that I found while doing a Google Images search. The song is one that I wrote/recorded back in the summer of 1999....

Thank you for sharing your life experiences here on YouTube!! Peace & Many Blessings,

Steve (phemohilia)

Many things...

Hi mike, just sending you a message saying your videos are just awesome i drink tea and one of my aunts and uncles are vegans. This makes me think and eat healthier. But any ways about the tea if it says natural is that "organic" well anyways after the stuff i got is gone I'm getting loose leaf and organic because i have Lipton tea. Just keep making videos HUGE help and gives me motivation to make those things. Also maybe make more tea videos
i love watchin them keep on rocking.

,Peace, jcharbaugh
(pronunciation: j, c, harbo)

hi

Hey mike I love all your videos they been helping with my troubles in my life. But recently I been suicidal you're the only person i have in my life, can you please help me.

Need Advice ^-^

hey mike how's it going love your videos, the reason for this message if mostly for my dad and a lil bit about me, 1 week ago we saw your how to lower your cholesterol video and we found it very useful and informative because my father was told by the doctor that he has high cholesterol he is 48 years old and rather new at trying to watch what he eats, he is very energetic and exercises frequently, i was wondering if you knew any other foods he can eat other than the ones you mentioned in your video and what he can do to watch his cholesterol level and how to measure the cholesterol intake he consumes, we tried asking his doctor but his doctor in my opinion is a nut job lol anywho it would help us a lot if you can help in anyway as far as information , since my father has high cholesterol then i may have the same problem in the future since i think it has been in the family since my great grandpa. If you have any websites or anything, any information would help!

Thank you mike and keep the videos rollin!
P.S shave that beard =P

Thanks.

Just wanted to thank you for all the time and effort you put into your videos, the site, and everything. I've learned a lot from watching, and can't wait for more.

You've truly been an inspiration, and thanks.

-Jeff-

Hey Mike :)

Hello Mike. My name is Elin and I'm a 22 year old girl from Norway. I have been struggling with weight loss until I saw your videos. Of course I have been trying to lose the weight for many years..since I was 17 I think (gained it all in Jr high as a result of some very bad years) but I never had any system in it and often I would eat too little and just gain it back when I started eating "normally" again. But now I feel like I have a plan that will work. Eating 1500 calories a day and burning 2000 or 2500 calories a day, and FIBER ;-). So I just want to thank you so much for your wonderful advice and videos. I love them and get so much inspiration and hope from lhem. I think my highest weight was 198 pounds and I am now 187 pounds and well on my way. Please don't ever stop making your videos and inspiring people all over the world!

Peace,
Elin

Hi there,
thank you a lot for your inspiration. I often eat quinoa now and wouldn t come to that without your inspiration. And it's a fantastic food. It tastes better than rice couscous and so on. I love mixing with tomatoes and so on (sorry for my bad English)

I love sushi, but i don't know if it's allowed to eat that as a vegetarian.

Greets nice,
Thomas

Love your videos

Hi there live life. I really enjoy your YouTube videos. I was very fascinated by your ability to floss so quickly. I have not mastered flossing that quickly and efficiently YET. I also watched your video about your teas. I love teas. In fact I became a kettle freak and did hours of research on kettles and finally found what I consider to be the best kettle on the planet in terms of non-toxic eco-friendly material. I also consume a particular very special tea that is not really a tea from the Amazon rainforest that is highly anti-fungal, anti-bacterial, anti-fungal and anti-inflammatory. In any case, I'd love to connect with you and become your friend. Please feel free to add me on Facebook so we can stay in touch,

With heart centered kindness,
Issac Ben-Avram

Hey Mike,

it may sound oh so very cliché, but you are really like an angel i think, sent from heaven... there aren't many people in the world like you, but having you in it makes life worth living! Watching your videos today have really inspired me. I was (literally) praying that someone would come along in my life to help me at the moment, so it´s all very odd (but good!)

When do you think your website will be up and running again? I need to make some changes in my life but in some ways i am scared to change, my bad habits are like my crutch... what would i do without that?

My problem is that i find it hard to deal with stress and negative emotions so i tend to comfort eat when i am feeling low... also I find it hard when i am in a situation whether at work or with friends, to say no to things... I feel awkward if i get annoyed about something, and i don't understand this... I guess I lack assertion at times... (Not always). If I was still living in England i would go see a counselor but living on this small island off the west coast of Africa, there isn't the variety or anyone professional who speaks English.

I do have to give myself a bit pat on the back though because I´ve got through a lot of hurdles in my life: bulimia, depression (due to many reasons, including my parents break up at 15, which changed my life and lead me onto a path that i hadn't envisaged career wise) and recently after ten years have managed to wean myself off anti-depressants (wey hey I am now 9 months meds free!!) and made the decision to break up from a negative relationship just four months ago, after 4 years of being together. I am now living on my own, the first time in my life... that´s taken some getting used to... but i have my faithful friend in tow, my cat, Jack... who will be 12 this year... I am 36.

So now, I want to lose ten pounds so i feel lighter and better in myself... but, like i said, i do tend to over eat when i am low or have had a bad day... yeah its definitely my reaction to negativity...do you have any advice on that? I do exercise regularly... i have to be careful though not to do too much cos of my days when i was v unbalanced, and would over exercise,... I also want to get my confidence back after a very damaging relationship.

Any advice would really really help... even if it's just a few words..... You really are an inspiration to me, and you wife is a very lucky lady!!! Incidentally, do you have any videos with her in it? Would be nice to see her. Do you have any children and pets???

So I send you kind wishes from the island of Fuerteventura, and truly hope you might reply to me.

Until then,

Claire xxx

Thanks

Just wanted to let you know that because of you i bought kiwi and quinoa my last trip to the grocery store lol. I looked at them while shopping but never picked em up so thanks to you i tried something new. I'm loving the kiwi, i eat it with the skin like i saw you did, it's pretty good.

Thanks again and keep the vids coming
xoxo
Shyla

wildcatsthree said...

> What a wonderful story; it brought tears to my eyes. I believe those kinds of things do happen, as our loved ones that have passed are always watching over us from above. And the fact that both fathers had flown jets is just too much of a coincidence.

PaulsHealthBlog.com said...

Great story, and yes, your father was at that wedding. You are his son, his blood. You thought of him at the right exact moment for a reason.

This post was well written. Thanks for sharing.

P.S. My father died of cancer too, after being on oxygen for eight long years.

He was an ex-smoker and did not take care of himself. It came back to get him in the end.

Urban Panther said...

My sister died at the age of 21. Sadly, my dad was the only one able to attend the funeral (long story). My sister was adopted. She was full Chippewa. As my dad was driving away from the funeral, on a long lonely stretch of British Columbia highway, a crow flew right in front of him, down the centre lane for a substantial period of time (much longer than normal bird behavior). My dad KNEW it was my sister.

Thanks for sharing that. It was a beautiful story.

M.d Tabish Faraz said...

As a heavy smoker myself who has started to think of quitting, I find myself more determent of quitting smoking after reading this beautiful post.

Let me tell you that this particular post has multiple levels of depths in it which reflects the brilliant talent of the writer. I absolutely loved the true story. Many thanks for sharing it, mate.

Hey Mike!
It's very appreciated that you give me the opportunity to send you messages directly. Like I said to my girlfriend COOL! Mike foster is my friend LOL Don't worry I'm not crazy, I'm just happy that you actually care about my life change. So here it is:
The past few years were the most difficult of my life. (up to now) I've quit smoking cigarettes (3years now) and since February 17th I've quit smoking pot. (Hardest ever) At first I was 205 pounds, which wasn't bad for a guy my size. Unfortunately, missing my smoking habits I started eating like a pig. And when I say like a pig, I mean crazy eating. When I was alone I could eat a whole pound of of bacon or 4 burgers from McDonald's. Something was missing in my life. I went up to 260 pounds in about 6 months. My doctor told me my pressure went up like crazy and that I had to do something before it was too late. (A lot of cardiacs in my family) That's when I started looking for help on the net. My first step was to go on YouTube where I found tons of videos on healthy life skills. But most of them were about products like fat burners and expensive programs. Then from a colleague at work I heard about the benefits of green tea and fat loss so i did a research on it. That's where I found livelife365 or should I say You. I watch your green tea video...the next day I was at the local health store and I bought an organic green tea and I fell in love with it. Then I started to watch you other videos about health, fat loss, balance and all your funny stuff to. Your ways had helped me very much. Your just so natural and if I may, you are not full of shit talk like all the folks trying to sell their body hurting products...I just love the fact that everything you do is natural. I've been doin' everything you recommend for three months now and.....I lost 18 pounds, regained focus and energy. I eat my banana apple oatmeal and ....for sure....my almonds every day. I'm not completely veggie but
Ived reduced a lot my meat eating to only chicken and fish. I am improving every day and I love it. Thanks to your advice my life is worth living 365 days a year. THANK YOU FOR EVERYTHING!

PEACE!!
Pierre Charbonneau

Mike,
It is my humble opinion that livelife365.com is a wonderful idea and is well worth the time and efforts you are giving to it. In my visit to your website I have enjoyed every video that I have viewed, and in each case I have gained something very positive from having viewed them.
I believe that we have all experienced times when we have needed some

guidance and/or direction in our lives and sometimes good sources for this can be limited or completely unavailable for some. You seem to offer what is needed and helpful to anyone seeking to become informed on a particular issue or concern that they may have.

I also believe that your decision to present your thoughts and ideas through video rather than in writing is appealing. It is a refreshing, and much needed, break from the endless blogs and various other web pages that sometimes seem only to be carbon copies of one another, and all too often they can be very boring and full of useless nonsense. I would say I have found this to not be the case when perusing through your video archives, but instead have found a treasure trove of good things in your generous offerings of sound advice.

You have inspired me Mike! Thank you!

Very humbly,

Daniel

Catatonic Kid said...

> Fantastic idea, Mike! Bring on the tasty goodness. You know for the marinara one thing I also like to add is a couple of bay leaves. They bring together all the other flavors and really make the whole thing pop.
>
> I eat meat twice a week and the rest is all veg so if you can come up with some satisfying takes on the comfort classics I'd be very excited.
>
> I much prefer the healthier option as I'm strict about sodium intake but finding truly tasty recipes not based on saturated fats to substitute for minimal salt is very difficult.

Robin Easton said...

> Cool Mike, you cook like ME!! How fun to see this. I love this idea. Good for you!!

Have you ever made vegetarian meatloaf, even my husband will eat it. I use pre-cooked brown rice, lentils, any other beans, onions, garlic, celery, (grated carrot or other veggies optional), a bit of whole grain flower, cayenne pepper to taste, etc. and bake it in a glass cake pan. I sometimes top it with tomato sauce that I make like your marinara sauce, which can be put on before baking so it seeps in.

You can also had whole oats to make it a bit stiffer.

This can also be made into veggie burgers. Sometimes I add rosemary and sage or try other herbs. I also pre-form the veggie burgers and freeze them cooked or uncooked...makes for quicker meals.

This is very fun what you are doing with these videos. Good job! And very inspiring for me. You're a natural! :):) Robin

Dori said...

Mike,
I'm a few days late to this post, but I just wanted to send my condolences about your stepfather. And also I wanted to thank you for such an insightful post about 2008. You are so right...we have to live life 365.

Mike, your blog videos are like a weekly presidential address to the nation!

Seriously, these are all good suggestions, especially one as simple as making sure to wash your hands. That alone goes a long way to prevent sickness during the winter time.

Thanks, Paul...

Martin in Bulgaria said...

You are a knight in shining armor to many with your blog Mike. I must admit I do most of those things you suggest anyway, in fact that's why I like winter, and it gives you reasons to do things. By the way, never had the flu or colds for years here, so I save on tissue paper.

Summer is more of a problem with over eating and just sitting around - it's too hot to do anything. Bit of a flip side of the coin there really.
Back on track - So glad I subscribed to your blog so I don't miss anything! Recommend others do this! Rock on Winter!

LisaNewton said...

I have a weakness for all of the above. It's sometimes very hard to say no, but now it must be.

Your quote, "Exercise control, control your weaknesses, and your weaknesses will become your strengths."

Love, love, love this. It's so true. If you're able to control your weaknesses, you'll slowly build self-esteem, which will lead to so many good things.

You've definitely got the answer here, Mike...............:)

Great post Mike!!! :-)

What an uplifting message and bravo to Pierre! Mike you do such great work here and you always inspire me to live a much healthier lifestyle. Keep up the great work ☺

Wow - I love the post, the message, the Pierre story, your song, and most of all YOU! How inspiring. One thing you said about hope really struck a chord -"we create hope". Yes, we are so capable of creating it! And with it, many things are created.

Like you, I have seen such joy and hope in the faces of the most unlikely people and places on this planet of ours. Sometimes it is ALL these people have and yet their hope outshines so many of us.

Thank you - again - for being you.
suZen

Andrea said...

> I was quite moved by this post and not because I related so well to your publishing woes (I recently had my first agent rejection, not to mention other story rejections in the past) but because I often have to struggle to find that glimmer of hope. But you hit it on the head: if those people who have it so much harder that they have every reason to give up...if they can hang in there and keep it moving, I have no reason whatsoever to whine or complain, especially since my life, relatively speaking, is pretty good. Thanks for the reminder, Mike.

Kathy said...

> Great stuff here. Watched the "lose 2 lbs/week" video. I know I'm doing that now (started Weight Watchers), but I hadn't really thought about the importance of fiber. I'm looking at labels more and more now, trying to find foods with more fiber. Thanks for the pep talk. My goal is to lose 30lbs by mid-summer. The thing I have to remember is that I didn't put the weight on quickly, so it can't come off quickly. Two pounds a week is doable and healthier. Thanks again, Mike…

I just love love love cherries. I've not had any yet this year, so now I am craving them. I did not know all the benefits of cherries. I mean I knew they were healthy but did not know about the melatonin/sleep thing. Now, I HAVE to go buy some.

Watching you eat them is making me go berserk. I'm sitting looking at the clock typing as fast as I can to get this done and see if I can get to the health food store and grab some cherries before it closes. You think I'm kidding, NOT!!! LOLOL!!!

Love this post and the vid. This is SUCH a cool site. I always want to eat whatever you are talking about!!! Thank you mike. Catch you later, I'm off to find some cherries. I've simply CRAVING them now. Hugs, Robin :))

Hi Mike!
Another dy-no-mite post! I think you have the gift to motivate a ROCK!

You know one thing you said at the beginning is something that makes me NUTS - people who say they don't have the time! I know so many folks ask me ALL the time, "How do you find the time to do so much?" It's not TIME that is lost here. It's that lack of wanting to do things you so eloquently spoke of - time is here and now, not lost. It's the people's lack of desire that is lost.

Thank you so so much for being such a bright beacon of light! Every visit here is a delight!

Lisa said...

I loved how you mentioned that it is a choice to see the bowl half empty or full. There are so many things out of our control, but how we view the world is in our control & has a huge effect on our happiness! Thanks for another great article!

Dr. Jarret Morrow said...

> Mike, another great post! I read your interview on Dr. Nicole's site.
> Most American's don't consume enough fiber. As you know,
> adequate fiber intake prevents not only constipation and obesity, but
> may also prevent heart disease, diabetes, and cancer.

This was a great video. I deal with A LOT of negativity in my life and in
fact I myself can be made to be quite negative and defeatist. It was
refreshing to hear the message in this video, I have watched several of your
videos and you really have something to say, I subscribed. Thanks

nls8520

I LOVE watching ur videos... U ARE SUCH A NATURAL! THANKS
FOR SHARING, BROTHER!

lakotasue

Thank you for this , I absolutely love watching your videos, because
you always have a story and you always tell it well !!!

xgirl2740Â

Yo this video was awesome.. Wish i could have the opportunity to meet you
1 day... good spirit man... def gonna check out some more of your videos...
and i actually bought an avocado today and didn't know how to eat it so
that's how i found your video. By the way it was delicious!!

Theratinthehouse

Mike, I'm 13 yrs. old I weighed a lot. Everyone at school made fun of me
last year and when i came back to school after a summer on your plan,
amazed everyone. They were shocked. No one has made fun of me since.
You even helped me get a girlfriend (my first due to my weight). You are a

great person. I thank you so much for changing my life. I hope you realize how grateful I am.

cornsnake1fan

Mike I want to thank you because I watched one of your other videos about how to lose weight and it has changed my life style. You inspired me to change the way I eat and think about food. So far I have lost 7 pounds with healthy eating and exercising in a month. To me that is a lot! It's like I have found the secret to losing weight. Thanks again

sweettangell41

Mike you totally rock!

I've learned that most diets work for the first 2 weeks because they almost always suggest you drink tons of water) Of course, it's water weight, but it's still weight right! LOL

I've got to get back to my weight lifting. I've been slacking the last few months.

You can burn 40% more if you stand up and watch your video:oP

Thanks for a great motivating video!

Zoeebella

Great Video. I am only 18 and I enjoy learning from you. All your videos are great keep the good work up. You have inspired me to live better. I am sure I am not the only one who is inspired by you. God bless and take care.

-Marwin Garmendia

I have visited many, many sites and I have to say that I am very impressed with your vision. I love your site! Mark S.

That's quite a website you have, Mike. Nice job! Do me a favor and keep the humor going. It's great. :)

Peace,
Michael

You know i really like this vid, I'm over weight (O-beast). I have it in my mind that i wana Lose weight and i find it hard to, even though i know it's possible, losing weight would be the best thing to ever happen to me. You give really good points on how to stop Obesity.

HULK91X16

You have a very soothing voice and if there's anyone I want to listen to, as far as my obesity, it's you. Thank you for taking the time out to speak to the world and motivate us who are trapped in bodies that may be alien to us. I am 4'10" and weigh 205 lbs. My body shut down after having my last child and my weight snuck up being me. I will continue to listen to your advice and hope to give you some feedback soon. MrJayoly

I used to drink coffee and eat very little fiber, then I viewed this video and your Green Tea video, and after a couple of weeks of replacing coffee with green tea, and sugar cereals with all bran and wheat flakes...I'm really feeling the difference...I have more energy, I'm not fatigued, I feel good.......I really enjoy your videos...keep up the good work.

HighOnMyOwnSupply

Mike this video, music and lyrics is probably one of the most creative video's I've ever watched on YT. I'm watching this with one big smile on my face. What you lack in hair, you make up with the better things that we only find inside ourselves. Thank you for bringing some warmth to my evening! Mark

If you think that I'm not gonna subscribe to your channel!! You are terribly wrong.

Been a long time since I have heard such an incredible video!!!

Boy!!! That was more than fun!!! It was truly fantastic my friend.

Congrats!!!! You deserve more stars that I can imagine******************************

bios36

i have to come and tell you that when I showed this song to my dad...he laughed so hard...LOL...he has been working a lot lately...and when he saw it he was really tired...and you still made him laugh...you rock!!! You should win an award for this and should be on the radio!!! Love you lots and lots!

bear6120

I love how enthusiastic and full of energy he is. That in itself is a great promotion for these teas! :)

I've tried Rooibos and Green Tea. I felt great drinking green tea, but felt nothing from the rooibos...although it's the better tasting of the two.

wadehjb

Thank you so much for this video. I'm a 20 yr. old college student and I'm trying my best to change my eating habits for the better. Green tea has become my new obsession! It's begun to help me concentrate in school, helps me exercise and keeps me awake during the day. It's so nice to have that healthy pick-me-up instead of settling for those energy drinks that make me crash. You're awesome! <3

ShadowedVeil7

You have really helped me a lot, you are an inspiration sir, god
bless and take care.

Peace

sechadyl

I LOVE your videos, you're very easy to watch. How do you know all this
information? At first I thought you were a chef, but then I realized you
know more about the body than a chef would. I am thinking a doctor of
some sort. You are going to get my family to visit the produce section for
more than apples and bananas. There are so many fruits and vegetables that
I would like to try, but I don't know how to prepare and eat them. I am glad
I found your videos.

OUWATZAHLE08

mike thx you bottom my heart love your work your like the second father to
me when i feel down i watch your videos and makes me feel better thx
again :)

samhamels

Love your videos man, keep it up! As a 19 year old person I'm always searching for new mentors, it seems like you are now one of them. I'm fascinated by all your 'life-wisdoms' and hope I'm able to incorporate them into my life. Thanks man :) really

Krain420

I absolutely love your videos Mike; so formal, straight to the point, and easy to understand/apply to daily life. I look forward to each one each week and I admire you greatly as a mentor and adviser. Keep up the good work!

Hi Mike,

Was browsing various tea videos and came across your site. I've watched a few of your videos but wanted to send you a direct message and let you know that I think what you're doing is awesome. Positive thinking and staying healthy is pretty hard these days, so it's cool to see someone spreading the message in their own way.

Do you write your stuff, or do you just go with it? I'm just getting into recording my own tea videos for Adagio and was curious as to whether you had any feedback on them. Care to check them out and let me know? I don't write anything and just come up with the basics on the spot, but it's to my detriment sometimes. You seem to have a steady train of thought when speaking on-camera, and was wondering if you had any insight on that.

Well, keep on keepin' on.

Thanks again.
-Trevor

Another excellent video and i know exactly how this relates to weight loss.

At age 22(about to turn 23) I tipped in at 297 lbs. at 6" 1

This was 4 months ago, Right now my current weight is 272 from eating right, exercising and from your videos, Mike.. I controlled the challenge. I took the problem by its balls. All the laziness and heavy eating habits the past 5 years took its toll on my body, but I made an initiative to get the weight off and never reach above 300 lb.

thx again Mike

BIGDADDYF50

And lastly, while I will always feel too young to be referred to as a grandfather:

Love these videos. It's sort of like getting advice from the grandfather I never had. good stuff Mike.

nls8520

All of the above comments are from my websites and YouTube. They are but a few of thousands and thousands of people, like yourself, who have changed their lives for the better and reached out to share their story and message with me and others. Hope to hear from **YOU** soon.

peace,

Mike

livelife365

Made in the USA
Lexington, KY
21 May 2015